M000285401

DO ONE THING
EVERY DAY
TO SLEEP WELL
EVERY NIGHT

A Journal by

Sleep Is Your Superpower

Matthew Walker, TED Talk

The title of sleep scientist Dr. Matthew Walker's popular 2019 TED Talk says it all. Not only does sleep benefit your mood, alertness, attention span, and learning, it also protects you. Chronic sleep problems can lead to disease and accidents as well as lower your productivity. If you picked up this book, you may already be wondering how to get a better night's sleep

Scientists have done much research on sleep—how it works and doesn't work and how to foster it. Note the essential takeaways on the SLEEP BASICS pages throughout this book. This feature includes recommendations for the best sleep conditions—routines, naps, exercises, and diet, how to wind down mentally and physically, and even where to find expert advice. Later you can test yourself with a low-stress QUIZ (answers provided).

The overview is bolstered by specific DREAMY IDEAS (such as why to wear warm socks to bed) and a range of soporific activities (e.g., eating SLEEPY FOODS or reciting SLEEPY MANTRAS) and products (e.g., SLEEPY SCENTS or SLEEPY TEXTURES). You can also muse over the experiences and beliefs of writers, artists, scientists, musicians, wits, public figures, spiritual leaders, and celebrities, who have chased sleep through the ages—and then record your own. You may even want to try out some of their more offbeat solutions. In the feature HOW THEY [FAMOUS PEOPLE] SLEPT, for example, you will learn that the famed novelist Marcel Proust lined his bedroom with cork to block out sounds.

We strongly encourage you to be your own sleep scientist as you experiment with what you read here. After trying out each of the various recommendations, rate your sleep on a scale of 1 to 5 Z's. The cumulative result will be the most complete body of sleep research on the single most important subject—you! We hope that all of this data, from without and within, will set you up for regular 5-Z's nights.

You may want to begin with SLEEP BASICS, then flip through the other pages for information and activities that suit your needs or mood or pique your interest on any given night. Your first act, though, should be to find your sleep baseline on the survey below. Then, after 365 pages of *Do One Thing Every Day to Sleep Well Every Night*, review your sleep ratings at the bottoms of pages and fill out the same survey at the end of the book.

Meanwhile, in the words of Sir Walter Scott, "To all, to each, a fair good night."

DATE: ___ / ___ / ___

SLEEP SURVEY

Number of hours I sleep at night: _____

    Bedtime: _____

    Wake time: _____

Naps: ☐ yes ☐ no

    How many? _____

    Average length: _____

Dinner time: _____

Unplug time: _____

Ways I relax before sleep: _____

How well I sleep (rate in Z's): Z Z Z Z Z

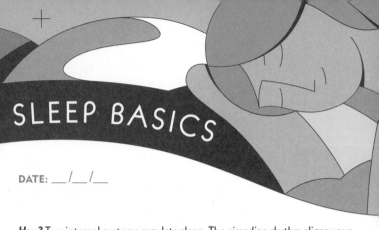

SLEEP BASICS

DATE: __ / __ / __

How? Two internal systems regulate sleep. The *circadian rhythm* aligns your daily waking and sleeping patterns to the 24-hour cycle of the day and night. The *sleep drive* gets stronger the longer you are awake. How much sleep you need depends on your age, according to the Centers for Disease Control and Prevention (CDC):

AGE GROUP	HOURS OF SLEEP
18–60 years	7 or more hours per night
61–64 years	7–9 hours
65 years and older	7–8 hours

Why? Sleep helps form and maintain pathways in the brain for learning and memory and helps you concentrate and respond quickly. It may also remove toxins in the brain and help process emotions.

I am _____ years old. I should sleep _____ hours nightly.

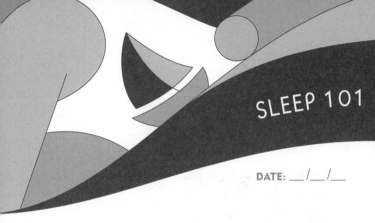

DATE: __/__/__

Sleep is not a single experience, but a cycle of two main stages: non-REM (rapid eye movement) sleep, which has three substages, and REM sleep. Your body moves through this sleep cycle about every 90 minutes.

Stage 1 (non-REM): Several minutes of light sleep. Heart rate, breathing, and eye movements are slow; muscles relax with occasional twitches.

Stage 2 (non-REM): Still light sleep, but heart rate and breathing slow and muscles relax even more; body temperature drops, eye movements stop.

Stage 3 (non-REM): Period of deep sleep needed to feel refreshed in the morning. Heart rate and breathing at lowest levels.

Stage 4 (REM): Eyes move rapidly under eyelids and brain waves are closer to wakefulness than in non-REM stages. Most dreams occur here.

I think I had REM sleep last night because:

_____

DATE: ___ /___ /___

Sleep that knits up the ravell'd sleave of care,

The death of each day's life, sore labour's bath,

Balm of hurt minds, great nature's second course,

Chief nourisher in life's feast.

William Shakespeare

What a good sleep does for me:

_____

_____

_____

_____

_____

Health is the first muse, and sleep is the condition to produce it.

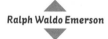

Ralph Waldo Emerson

How I feel healthier after last night's good sleep:

_____

_____

_____

_____

_____

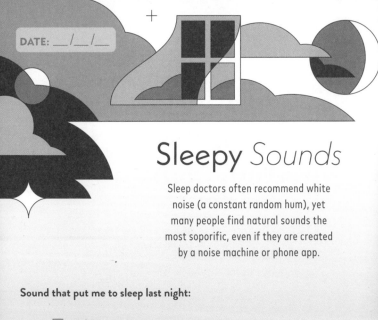

DATE: ___/___/___

Sleepy *Sounds*

Sleep doctors often recommend white noise (a constant random hum), yet many people find natural sounds the most soporific, even if they are created by a noise machine or phone app.

Sound that put me to sleep last night:

☐ rushing air

☐ ocean waves

☐ waterfall

☐ rain

☐ white noise

☐ _____
                      other

Rate sleep in Z's: Z Z Z Z Z

The rain plays a little sleep song on our roof at night.

Langston Hughes

Song from nature that put me to sleep last night:

_____

_____

_____

_____

_____

YOUR HAIR MAY
BE BRUSHED,
BUT YOUR MIND'S
UNTIDY.
YOU'VE HAD ABOUT
SEVEN HOURS' SLEEP
SINCE FRIDAY.

◆

Ogden Nash

DATE: ___ /___ /___

WHAT I FEEL LIKE AFTER THE WEEKEND WITH 7 HOURS' SLEEP SINCE FRIDAY:

_____

_____

_____

_____

_____

DATE: ___ /___ /___

WHAT I LOOK LIKE AFTER THE WEEKEND WITH 7 HOURS' SLEEP SINCE FRIDAY:

When action grows unprofitable, gather information; when information grows unprofitable, sleep.

Ursula K. Le Guin

Last night I knew it was time to go to sleep when doing this grew unprofitable:

_____

_____

Today I feel:

_____

_____

DATE: __ / __ / __

Dog-tiredness is such a lovely prayer, really, if only we would recognize it as such.

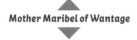

Mother Maribel of Wantage

Last night I kept on going even though I was dog-tired from doing this:

_____

_____

Today I feel:

_____

_____

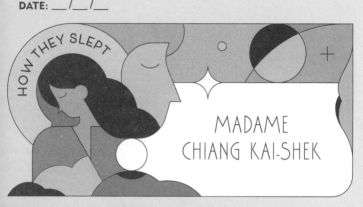

HOW THEY SLEPT

MADAME CHIANG KAI-SHEK

Former First Lady of the Republic of China, Madame Chiang Kai-Shek took her silk sheets with her everywhere, including to the White House.

What I bring with me to sleep in someone else's house:

_____

_____

_____

_____

_____

I always take a cashmere blanket and I have pictures of my family in my passport holder. I always go to sleep on the plane.

Kate Moss

What I need to sleep on a plane:

_____

_____

_____

_____

_____

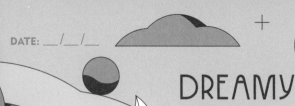

DATE: __/__/__

DREAMY IDEAS

The Bath Effect

A warm shower or bath an hour or two before bedtime can help you sleep more quickly and deeply. The warm water raises your skin temperature, causing your internal temperature to fall, a prelude to sleep. Some people add Epsom salts, which contain magnesium, a muscle relaxant.

Last night I took a warm ☐ bath ☐ shower before bedtime.

Rate sleep in Z's: Z Z Z Z Z

A hot bath! How exquisite a vespertine pleasure, how luxurious, fervid and flagrant a consolation for the rigours, the austerities, the renunciations of the day.

Rose Macaulay

After a hard day, last night's luxurious bath readied me for a consoling sleep. This morning I feel:

_____

_____

_____

_____

_____

DATE: __ / __ / __

SENSELESS THOUGHT I HAD LAST NIGHT:

_____

_____

_____

_____

_____

_____

DATE: __ / __ / __

REMOTE SOURCE OF A THOUGHT FROM LAST NIGHT:

_____

_____

_____

_____

_____

_____

BEWARE THOUGHTS THAT COME IN THE NIGHT. THEY AREN'T TURNED PROPERLY; THEY COME IN ASKEW, FREE OF SENSE AND RESTRICTION, DERIVING FROM THE MOST REMOTE OF SOURCES.

William Least Heat-Moon

I DREAM A LOT. I DO MORE PAINTING WHEN I'M NOT PAINTING. IT'S IN THE SUBCONSCIOUS.

Andrew Wyeth

What I created in my subconscious last night:

_____

_____

_____

_____

_____

We sleep, but the loom of life never stops and the pattern which was weaving when the sun went down is weaving when it comes up tomorrow.

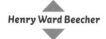

Henry Ward Beecher

What I accomplished in my sleep last night:

_____

_____

_____

_____

_____

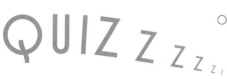
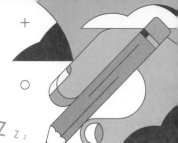

QUIZ zzz

Sleep Facts

True or False?

1. People often get less sleep as they get older.   T   F

2. Everyone needs 8 hours of sleep.   T   F

3. You can catch up on lost sleep on the weekends.   T   F

4. Watching TV helps you fall asleep.   T   F

5. People who exercise regularly during the day tend   T   F
   to sleep better.

6. Going to bed hungry or with a full stomach   T   F
   impedes sleep.

7. Alcohol helps you sleep.   T   F

Answers: 1, 5, and 6 are True.

I woke up one morning, [my girlfriend] asked me if I slept good. I said, "No, I made a few mistakes."

Steven Wright

Did you sleep good?

☐ Yes!

☐ No, I made a few mistakes:

_____

_____

_____

The amount of sleep required by the average person is about five minutes more.

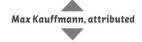

Max Kauffmann, attributed

I need _____ + 5 minutes of sleep every night.

Happiness is waking up, looking at the clock, and finding that you still have two hours left to sleep.

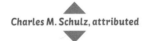

Charles M. Schulz, attributed

This morning I got up at _____, looked at the clock, and went back to sleep. Ahhhh!

AND I STILL REMEMBER IT THAT OF ALL THE NIGHTS THAT EVER I SLEPT IN MY LIFE, I NEVER DID PASS A NIGHT WITH MORE EPICURISM OF SLEEP.

Samuel Pepys

DATE: ___ /___ /___

THE NIGHT I PASSED WITH THE MOST EPICURISM OF SLEEP:

_____

_____

WHY:

_____

_____

DATE: ___ /___ /___

THE NIGHT I PASSED WITH THE LEAST EPICURISM OF SLEEP:

_____

_____

WHY:

_____

_____

If I had slept, I should not know so well the poets.

Eliza Boyle O'Reilly

If I had slept last night, I wouldn't know this:

_____

_____

_____

_____

_____

I have benevolent insomnia. I wake up, and my mind is preternaturally clear. The world is quiet. I can read or write. It seems like stolen time. It seems like I have a twenty-eight-hour day.

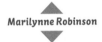

Marilynne Robinson

If I had slept last night, I wouldn't have done this:

_____

_____

_____

_____

_____

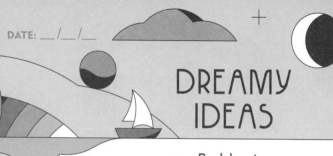

DREAMY IDEAS

Bedsheets

Many people believe that sheets with the highest thread counts (the number of horizontal and vertical threads per inch) are the softest. Some bedding experts, however, recommend choosing sheets made from the highest-quality cotton instead—long-staple or extra-long-staple threads.

Today I went to a shop and tested cotton sheets. These were the softest:

_____

thread count: _____

cotton quality: _____

The cool kindliness of sheets, that soon Smooth away trouble.

Rupert Brooke

Kind of sheets on my bed:

_____

_____

How they make me feel:

_____

_____

Sleep is the best (and easiest) creative aphrodisiac.

Debbie Millman

A creative idea aroused by my sleep last night:

_____

_____

_____

_____

_____

Even a soul submerged in sleep is hard at work and helps make something of the world.

Heraclitus

A useful idea worked out in my sleep:

_____

_____

_____

_____

_____

DATE: ___ / ___ / ___

A NEW SIGN OF HEALTH IN MY BODY AFTER LAST NIGHT'S GOOD SLEEP:

_____

_____

_____

_____

_____

DATE: ___ / ___ / ___

A NEW SIGN OF HEALTH IN MY MIND AFTER LAST NIGHT'S GOOD SLEEP:

_____

_____

_____

_____

_____

The beginning of health is sleep.

Irish proverb

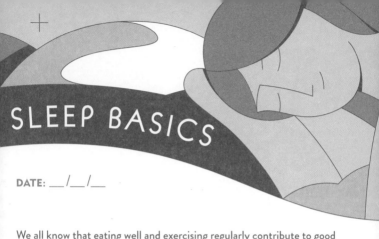

SLEEP BASICS

DATE: ___ / ___ / ___

We all know that eating well and exercising regularly contribute to good health. But a healthy lifestyle also contributes to good sleep. The food plan from the National Institutes of Health (NIH) recommends a variety of vegetables and whole fruits; a variety of proteins; half of your grains to be whole grains; fat-free or low-fat dairy products; and no added sugar, saturated fat, or salt.

Reminders: 1) Finish dinner at least 2 hours before bedtime to allow for digestion. 2) Avoid too many fluids to reduce the need to get up and urinate.

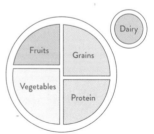

☐ Yesterday I followed the NIH advice.

Rate sleep in Z's: Z Z Z Z Z

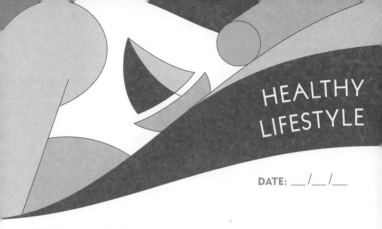

DATE: __ / __ / __

NIH Recommendations

Adults need at least 150 minutes of moderate-intensity exercise a week.
This should include muscle-strengthening exercises, such as doing push-
ups or lifting weights, at least 2 days a week.

Exercise Sleep Warning

Traditionally experts have advised ending your workout 2 to 3 hours before
bedtime. Exercise can stimulate the nervous system, increase heart rate,
and raise body temperature, all of which may interfere with sleep. New
research suggests, however, that only *high*-intensity exercise needs to stop
1 hour before bedtime. *What works for you? Be your own sleep researcher.*

☐ **Yesterday I exercised as the NIH recommends:**

Intensity level of my exercise: ☐ high   ☐ medium   ☐ low

Rate sleep in Z's: Z Z Z Z Z

As the night gets dark, let your worries fade. Sleep peacefully knowing you've done all you can do for today.

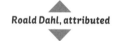

Roald Dahl, attributed

☐ I did all I could do for today. Good night.

DATE: __ / __ / __

Tired Nature's sweet restorer, balmy sleep!

Edward Young

After a balmy sleep, I woke restored, and today I can tackle this:

_____

_____

_____

_____

_____

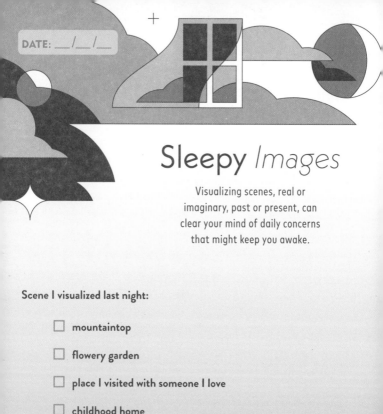

DATE: __/__/__

Sleepy *Images*

Visualizing scenes, real or
imaginary, past or present, can
clear your mind of daily concerns
that might keep you awake.

Scene I visualized last night:

☐ mountaintop

☐ flowery garden

☐ place I visited with someone I love

☐ childhood home

☐ beach vacation

☐ _____
　　　　　　　　　　other

Rate sleep in Z's: Z Z Z Z Z

DATE: __ / __ / __

Thank God I have the seeing eye, that is to say, as I lie in bed I can walk step by step on the fells and rough land seeing every stone and flower and patch of bog and cotton pass where my old legs will never take me again.

Beatrix Potter

Where my seeing eye led me before sleep last night:

_____

_____

_____

_____

_____

IT IS A COMMON
EXPERIENCE
THAT A PROBLEM
DIFFICULT AT NIGHT
IS RESOLVED IN THE
MORNING AFTER THE
COMMITTEE OF SLEEP
HAS WORKED ON IT.

John Steinbeck

DATE: __ / __ / __

PERSONAL PROBLEM THE COMMITTEE OF SLEEP RESOLVED LAST NIGHT:

_____

_____

_____

_____

_____

_____

DATE: __ / __ / __

PROFESSIONAL PROBLEM THE COMMITTEE OF SLEEP RESOLVED LAST NIGHT:

_____

_____

_____

_____

_____

_____

I don't need an alarm clock. My ideas wake me.

Ray Bradbury

The idea that woke me this morning:

_____

_____

_____

_____

DATE: __/__/__

I had one of those dreams when I was 23. When I suddenly woke up, I was thinking: what if we could download the whole web, and just keep the links and . . . . Amazingly, I had no thought of building a search engine [Google]. The idea wasn't even on the radar.

Larry Page

An off-the-radar idea that woke me up this morning:

_____

_____

_____

_____

_____

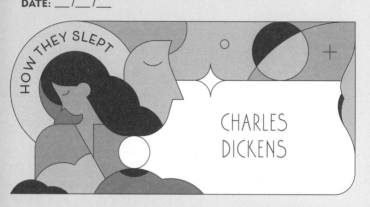

HOW THEY SLEPT

CHARLES DICKENS

The writer Charles Dickens moved his bed wherever he slept so that his head pointed north and his feet south. He thought that this would allow the earth's magnetic currents to flow correctly through his body.

Check one:

☐ Hogwash!

☐ The position of _____ in my bedroom helps me sleep better.

If you can't get to sleep, try lying on the end of the bed—you might drop off.

Anonymous

The position that helps me drop off to sleep:

_____

_____

_____

_____

_____

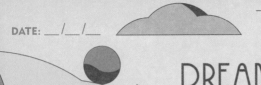

DREAMY IDEAS

Relaxing Breath

Repeating a "relaxing breath" can help you get to sleep by reducing anxiety. Some claim that this technique can work in a single minute.

1. Place your tongue on the roof of your mouth, just behind your teeth.

2. Breathe in for 4 seconds.

3. Hold the breath for 7 seconds.

4. Exhale for 8 seconds.

It worked in _____ minutes (I think).

Rate sleep in Z's: Z Z Z Z Z

There is no joy but calm!

Alfred, Lord Tennyson

How I achieved a joyous calm last night:

_____

_____

_____

_____

_____

DATE: ___ / ___ / ___

FRESH THOUGHT ON AWAKENING TODAY:

_____

_____

_____

_____

_____

_____

DATE: ___ / ___ / ___

SIGN OF JOYOUS HEALTH ON AWAKENING TODAY:

_____

_____

_____

_____

_____

_____

Come, blessed barrier between day and day, Dear mother of fresh thoughts and joyous health!

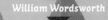

William Wordsworth

In sleep a king, but waking no such matter.

William Shakespeare

Who I was in my dream last night:

_____

_____

_____

_____

_____

Her face was veiled, yet to my fancied sight

Love, sweetness, goodness, in her person shined

So clear as in no face with more delight.

But, oh! as to embrace me she inclined,

I waked, she fled, and day brought back my night.

John Milton

My dream lover:

_____

_____

_____

_____

_____

QUIZ z z z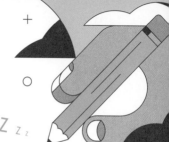

What to Do When You Can't Sleep

True or False?

1. Get out of bed.   T   F

2. Check email.   T   F

3. Read a b-o-r-i-n-g print book.   T   F

4. Watch a show on an electronic device.   T   F

5. Stay in bed and will yourself to sleep.   T   F

6. Do a mindless chore, then return to bed.   T   F

Answers: 1, 3, and 6 are True.

There are twelve hours in the day, and about fifty in the night.

Marie de Rabutin-Chantal, Marquise de Sévigné

Last night was 50 hours long because:

_____

_____

_____

_____

A nap, my friend, is a brief period of sleep which overtakes superannuated persons when they endeavour to entertain unwelcome visitors or to listen to scientific lectures.

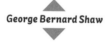

George Bernard Shaw

Why I napped today:

_____

_____

_____

_____

_____

I USUALLY TAKE A TWO-HOUR NAP FROM ONE TO FOUR.

Yogi Berra

Today I took a 20-minute nap (what most sleep experts advise)

from ____:____ to ____:____.

Afterward I felt _____.

I CAN NEVER DECIDE
WHETHER MY DREAMS
ARE THE RESULT OF
MY THOUGHTS, OR
MY THOUGHTS ARE THE
RESULT OF MY DREAMS.

D. H. Lawrence

DATE: ___/___/___

DREAM THAT WAS THE RESULT OF MY THOUGHTS:

_____

_____

_____

_____

_____

_____

DATE: ___/___/___

THOUGHT THAT WAS THE RESULT OF MY DREAM:

_____

_____

_____

_____

_____

DATE: ___ /___ /___

There is no place like a bed for confidential disclosures between friends. Man and wife, they say, there open the very bottom of their souls to each other; and some old couples often lie and chat over old times till nearly morning.

Herman Melville

Pillow talk last night:

_____

_____

_____

_____

_____

I did not sleep. I never do when I am over-happy, over-unhappy, or in bed with a strange man.

Edna O'Brien

I did not sleep last night because I was:

☐ over-happy

☐ over-unhappy

☐ in bed with a strange person

☐ _____
    other

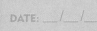

DREAMY IDEAS

Daylight Saving Time

Daylight saving time moves the clock 1 hour forward in the spring and back in the fall. It can disrupt your sleep/wake cycle for a few days or more.

The best solution is to adjust slowly, starting about a week in advance. Go to bed 10 to 15 minutes earlier or later than usual each night. If you decide instead to go cold turkey, the key is to avoid daytime naps of more than 20 minutes.

This year I:

☐ adjusted slowly and steadily to DST

☐ went cold turkey

Rate sleep in Z's: Z Z Z Z Z

In winter I get up at night,
And dress by yellow candle-light.
In summer, quite the other way,
I have to go to bed by day.

Robert Louis Stevenson

I am ☐ for ☐ against doing away with daylight saving time.

Snoring keeps the monsters away.

Judy Blume

Advantages of sleeping with a snorer:

☐ keeps the monsters away

☐ _____

☐ _____

☐ NONE!!

On his side of the bed Mr. Judson began to conduct a full-scale orchestra, and every instrument had sat out in the rain.

Dorothy West

Last night I tried to block the sound of my bedmate's snoring by:

- ☐ using a white-noise machine or phone app

- ☐ wearing earplugs

- ☐ asking the snorer to side-sleep

- ☐ exiling the snorer (no fun!)

- ☐ _____
     other

Rate sleep in Z's: Z Z Z Z Z

DATE: ___ / ___ / ___

HOW I FELT TODAY BECAUSE I WENT TO SLEEP AT THE WRONG TIME (___:___ .M.):

_____

_____

_____

_____

_____

_____

DATE: ___ / ___ / ___

HOW I FELT TODAY BECAUSE I OVERSLEPT UNTIL (___:___ .M.):

_____

_____

_____

_____

_____

Preserve me from unseasonable and immoderate sleep.

Samuel Johnson

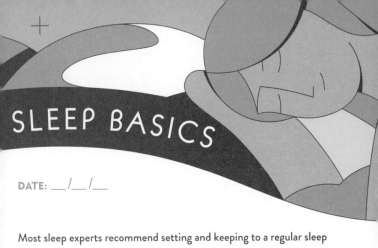

SLEEP BASICS

DATE: __/__/__

Most sleep experts recommend setting and keeping to a regular sleep schedule, going to sleep and getting up at the same times each day. Even on weekends, this schedule should not change by more than an hour. An unpredictable routine can disturb your circadian rhythm, your internal clock, confusing your body about whether to be asleep or awake. People with irregular schedules are more likely to develop symptoms of insomnia. They may have trouble falling asleep or staying asleep.

My ideal schedule:

Bedtime:

Wake-Up Time:

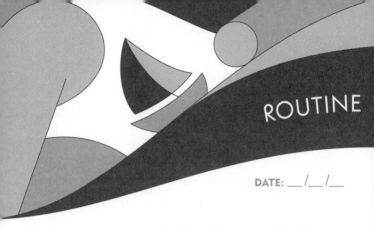

ROUTINE

DATE: __ / __ / __

Experts also recommend a predictable wind-down schedule of quiet, calming activities leading up to bedtime.

These calming activities are part of my ideal wind-down routine (number them in order):

_____ stating affirmations

_____ taking a warm bath

_____ slow breathing

_____ expressing gratitude

_____ meditating

_____ praying

_____ listening to soft music

_____ writing a plan for the morning

_____ stretching

_____ _____
                other

Rate sleep in Z's: Z Z Z Z Z

DATE: ___/___/___

I woke up with a lovely tune in my head
["Yesterday"]. I thought, "That's great, I wonder
what that is?" There was an upright piano
next to me, to the right of the bed by the
window. . . . I liked the melody a lot but because
I'd dreamed it I couldn't believe I'd written it.

Paul McCartney

I woke up and wrote down this great thing I dreamed:

_____

_____

_____

_____

_____

The old idea of a composer suddenly having a terrific idea and sitting up all night to write it is nonsense. Nighttime is for sleeping.

Benjamin Britten

After being fueled by a full night's sleep, this brilliant idea came to me today:

_____

_____

_____

_____

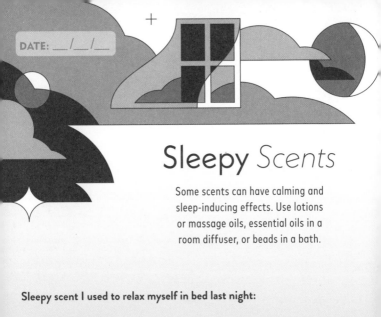

DATE: __ / __ / __

Sleepy *Scents*

Some scents can have calming and
sleep-inducing effects. Use lotions
or massage oils, essential oils in a
room diffuser, or beads in a bath.

Sleepy scent I used to relax myself in bed last night:

☐ lavender

☐ rose

☐ chamomile

☐ sweet marjoram

☐ bergamot

☐ _____
　　　　　　other

Rate sleep in Z's: Z Z Z Z Z

In the evening, I have a bath before bed; it's a ritual. I'm a bathing professional—I have different bubble baths, salts, beads, and oils.

Oprah Winfrey

I am a bathing ☐ amateur ☐ professional.

Sleepy scent I added to my bath last night:

_____

Rate sleep in Z's: Z Z Z Z Z

LET SLEEPING DOGS LIE.

Geoffrey Chaucer

DATE: ___/___/___

HOW I REACTED WHEN I WAS WAKENED FROM A DEEP SLEEP:

_____

_____

_____

_____

_____

_____

DATE: ___/___/___

HOW I REACTED WHEN I WOKE UP ON MY OWN AFTER A FULL SLEEP LAST NIGHT:

_____

_____

_____

_____

_____

DATE: ___/___/___

Never go to bed mad. Stay up and fight.

Phyllis Diller

—

Last night we resolved a disagreement about _____

and went to sleep.

Let's contend no more, Love,

Strive nor weep:

All be as before, Love,

—Only sleep!

Robert Browning

Last night we let sleep a disagreement about _____.

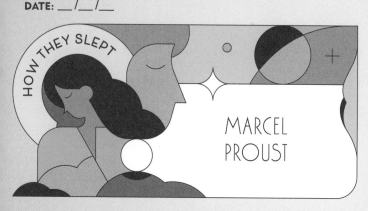

HOW THEY SLEPT

MARCEL PROUST

The writer Marcel Proust lined his bedroom with cork so that no sound could disturb his sleep.

How I block sound from my bedroom:

- ☐ white-noise machine
- ☐ fan
- ☐ air conditioner
- ☐ cork
- ☐ _____

        other

NOISE CREATES ILLUSIONS.
SILENCE BRINGS TRUTH.

Maxime Lagacé

Truth that came to me in the silence before sleep last night:

_____

_____

_____

_____

_____

_____

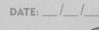

DREAMY IDEAS

Acupressure

There are many different points on your body where adding pressure can help you relax and sleep. One of them is just below the innermost part of your eyebrows. If you feel a small notch, you are in the right position. Place both thumbs there and, applying gentle pressure, move left and right.

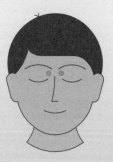

☐ **Did it!**

Rate sleep in Z's: Z Z Z Z Z

DATE: __ / __ / __

For every evil under the sun,
There is a remedy, or there is none.
If there be one, try and find it;
If there be none, never mind it.

Mother Goose

Last night I relaxed these points on my body by applying pressure here:

☐ inner leg, just above the ankle

☐ underside of the wrist

☐ base of the skull, right behind the ear

☐ top of foot, between the big toe and the second toe

Rate sleep in Z's: **Z Z Z Z Z**

DATE: ___ / ___ / ___

MY PERSONAL DARKNESS LAST NIGHT:

_____

_____

_____

_____

_____

_____

DATE: ___ / ___ / ___

MY PERFECT LIGHT THIS MORNING:

_____

_____

_____

_____

_____

THOUGH MY SOUL MAY SET IN DARKNESS, IT WILL RISE IN PERFECT LIGHT;

I HAVE LOVED THE STARS TOO TRULY TO BE FEARFUL OF THE NIGHT.

Sarah Williams

The recurrent dream. Mine is appearing before lecture audiences in my shirttail. A most disagreeable dream.

Mark Twain

A disagreeable, recurrent dream I had last night:

_____

_____

_____

_____

_____

DATE: ___/___/___

Have you noticed . . . there is never any third act in a nightmare? They bring you to a climax of terror and then leave you there. They are the work of poor dramatists.

Max Beerbohm

I woke from this nightmare last night before it was resolved:

_____

_____

_____

_____

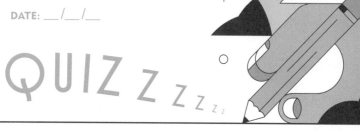

QUIZ Z z z z z

What's Wrong with This Bedroom for Sleep?

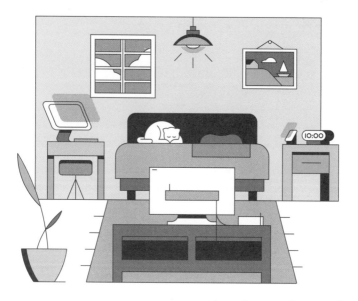

Answers: shadeless window, alarm clock facing bed, TV, computer on desk, cell phone on night table, light on, pet on bed

New Rule: Stop putting all those pillows on the bed. Attention, interior designers, hotel maids, and real housewives of New Jersey: It's a bed, not an obstacle course.

Bill Maher

I keep _____ pillows on my bed and have room to sleep.
       number

The last refuge of the insomniac
is a sense of superiority to the
sleeping world.

Leonard Cohen

Ha, sleepers! I may not have been able to sleep last night, but I got this

done while you were sacked out:

_____

_____

_____

_____

DATE: __ / __ / __

If a man had as many ideas during the day as he does when he has insomnia, he'd make a fortune.

Griff Niblack

I had _____ ideas last night when I couldn't sleep:
     number

_____

_____

_____

_____

_____

YOU ARE THE BIGGEST ENEMY OF YOUR OWN SLEEP.

Pawan Mishra

HOW I KNOWINGLY SABOTAGED MY SLEEP LAST NIGHT:

_____

_____

_____

_____

_____

_____

HOW I SABOTAGED MY SLEEP BY MISTAKE LAST NIGHT:

_____

_____

_____

_____

_____

_____

Try thinking of love, or something.
Amor vincit insomnia.
[Love conquers insomnia.]

Christopher Fry

Last night, thinking of _____ conquered my insomnia.

Sleep I can get nane,
For thinking on
my dearie.

Robert Burns

Sleep I can get nane, for thinking on _____.

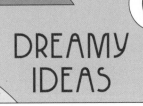

DREAMY IDEAS

Alcohol

Don't have more than two drinks at night, and stop drinking at least 3 hours before you go to sleep. Alcohol in your system can suppress REM sleep and wake you up.

☐ **Did it!**

Rate sleep in Z's: Z Z Z Z Z

R-E-M-O-R-S-E

Those dry Martinis did the work for me;
Last night at twelve I felt immense,
Today I feel like thirty cents.
My eyes are bleared, my coppers hot,
I'll try to eat, but I cannot.
It is no time for mirth and laughter;
The cold, gray dawn of the morning after.

George Ade

I drank too much too late last night. My morning after:

_____

_____

_____

_____

_____

DATE: __/__/__

The pillows are supposed to be pointed a certain way. The open side of the pillowcase is supposed to be pointed in toward the other side of the bed.

Stephen King

My bedtime ritual:

_____

_____

_____

_____

_____

The regularity of a habit is generally in proportion to its absurdity.

Marcel Proust

My most absurd bedtime ritual:

_____

_____

_____

_____

_____

DATE: ___ / ___ / ___

LAST NIGHT'S DREAM ABOUT SOMETHING I DIDN'T KNOW I KNEW:

_____

_____

_____

_____

_____

_____

DATE: ___ / ___ / ___

LAST NIGHT'S DREAM ABOUT SOMETHING I DID NOT KNOW:

_____

_____

_____

_____

_____

_____

Some dreams tell us what we wish to believe. Some dreams tell us what we fear. Some dreams are of what we know though we may not know we knew it. The rarest dream is the dream that tells us what we did not know.

Ursula K. Le Guin

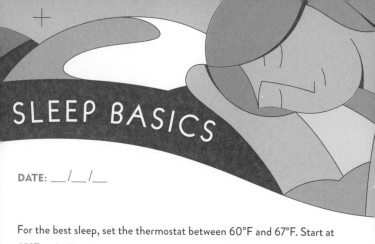

SLEEP BASICS

DATE: __/__/__

For the best sleep, set the thermostat between 60°F and 67°F. Start at 65°F and adjust the temperature up or down within that range until you are comfortable. The goal is to cool down your body's internal temperature by 2 to 3 degrees, enhancing the change that occurs naturally as you fall asleep. Too high or too low a temperature (above 75°F or below 54°F) can cause you to wake up.

My bedroom temperature last night: _____

☐ too hot ☐ too cold ☐ just right

Where I will set the thermostat tonight: _____

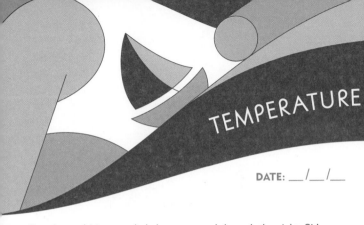

Two sleep positions can help keep you cool through the night. Side-sleepers have the least contact with the mattress. For back sleepers, the "starfish" position—arms and legs stretched out—allows air to circulate.

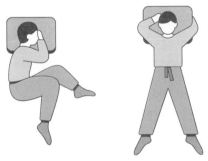

Last night I slept:

☐ on my side ☐ like a starfish ☐ _____
other

Rate sleep in Z's: Z Z Z Z Z

I lingered round them, under that benign sky: watched the moths fluttering among the heath and harebells, listened to the soft wind breathing through the grass, and wondered how anyone could ever imagine unquiet slumbers for the sleepers in that quiet earth.

Emily Brontë

Sights and sounds of the outdoors that help me sleep:

_____

_____

_____

_____

_____

Nothing can beat the smell of dew and flowers and the odor that comes out of the earth when the sun goes down.

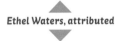

Ethel Waters, attributed

Smells of the outdoors that help me sleep:

_____

_____

_____

_____

_____

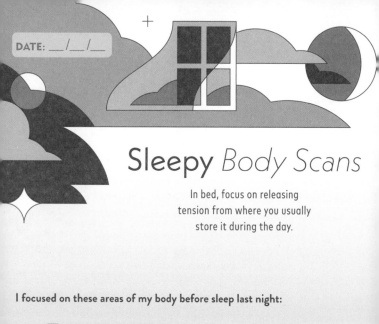

DATE: ___/___/___

Sleepy *Body Scans*

In bed, focus on releasing
tension from where you usually
store it during the day.

I focused on these areas of my body before sleep last night:

☐ face (begin with the scalp, then eyes, ears, mouth, jaw)

☐ neck (rotate your neck until you find a comfortable position)

☐ shoulders (lower shoulders; relax arms, hands, fingers)

☐ chest (take a deep breath in through your nose and out

through your mouth; repeat as needed)

☐ _____

other

Rate sleep in Z's: Z Z Z Z Z

DATE: __ / __ / __

There was no reality to pain
when it left one, though
when it held one fast all
other realities faded.

Rachel Field

How I felt when the tension left my _____:

_____

_____

_____

_____

_____

WHATEVER GETS YOU THRU THE NIGHT

John Lennon

DATE: __ / __ / __

A NEW SLEEP STRATEGY I TRIED LAST NIGHT:

_____

_____

_____

_____

Rate sleep in Z's: Z Z Z Z Z

DATE: __ / __ / __

A TWEAK OF AN OLD SLEEP STRATEGY I TRIED LAST NIGHT:

_____

_____

_____

_____

Rate sleep in Z's: Z Z Z Z Z

It appears that every man's insomnia is as different from his neighbor's as are their daytime hopes and aspirations.

F. Scott Fitzgerald

Describe your friend's insomnia:

_____

_____

Describe your particular insomnia:

_____

_____

DATE: __ /__ /__

[I] kept falling in and out of it [sleep] like out of a boat or a tipping hammock.

Rose Tremain

Last night I kept falling in and out of sleep like _____.

_____

_____

_____

_____

_____

DATE: __ / __ / __

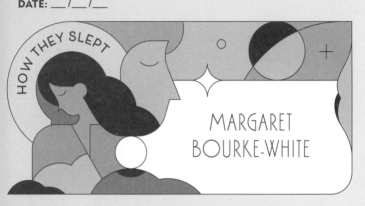

HOW THEY SLEPT

MARGARET BOURKE-WHITE

Photojournalist Margaret Bourke-White loved sleeping and writing outdoors in a contraption she made that could be rolled to different parts of her property. She went to bed at 8:00 P.M., woke at 4:00 A.M., and began writing just before daylight.

My experience sleeping outdoors: ☐ in a tent ☐ in a hammock

☐ on the beach ☐ _____
                                          other

_____

_____

_____

_____

By the time the sun rose, I was sealed in my own planet and safe from the distractions of the day.

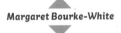

Margaret Bourke-White

How a good sleep protects me from the distractions of the day:

_____

_____

_____

_____

_____

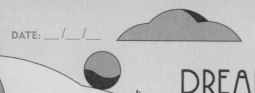

DATE: __/__/__

DREAMY IDEAS

Don't Stay in Bed

If you are lying in bed for 20 to 25 minutes and can't fall asleep, or if you awaken and can't fall back asleep, get up and do something quiet and boring in another room. Sit in a comfortable chair and listen to gentle music or a recorded book, read with dimmed lights, draw, fold laundry, knit—nothing mentally stressful or related to work. And do not return to the bedroom until you feel sleepy.

Last night I followed this advice until I felt sleepy:

_____

_____

Rate sleep in Z's: Z Z Z Z Z

You would never sit at the dinner table waiting to get hungry. So why would you lie in bed waiting to get sleepy?

Matthew Walker

Last night, when I couldn't sleep, I sat in the _____ and
room

_____ for _____ until I felt sleepy.
did what?   how long?

DATE: ___ / ___ / ___

A PHYSICAL PAIN SLEEP MUFFLED LAST NIGHT:

_____

_____

_____

_____

_____

_____

DATE: ___ / ___ / ___

A PAINFUL THOUGHT SLEEP MUFFLED LAST NIGHT:

_____

_____

_____

_____

_____

I REACHED FOR
SLEEP AND DREW IT
ROUND ME LIKE A
BLANKET MUFFLING
PAIN AND THOUGHT
TOGETHER IN THE
MERCIFUL DARK.

Mary Stewart

O God! I could be bounded in a nutshell, and count myself a king of infinite space, were it not that I have bad dreams.

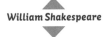

William Shakespeare

My bad dream last night:

_____

_____

_____

_____

_____

_____

Her lips were red, her looks were free,
Her locks were yellow as gold:
Her skin was white as leprosy,
The Night-mare Life-in-Death was she,
Who thicks man's blood with cold.

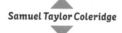

Samuel Taylor Coleridge

Draw an image from your nightmare last night.

DATE: __/__/__

QUIZ z z z _z

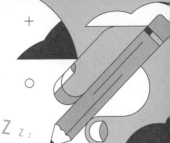

Foods to Avoid Before Going to Bed

Find the six unhelpful night foods in this puzzle. Words can go in any direction and can share letters if they cross. NOTE: Don't be fooled by the four soporific foods in here.

```
P  E  S  E  E  H  C  C  C  S
S  D  O  F  Y  J  H  H  S  I
M  D  E  A  G  D  O  I  T  W
L  Z  N  P  T  C  G  P  E  I
E  E  I  O  O  M  U  S  A  K
T  E  I  L  M  D  E  R  K  K
M  M  A  G  D  L  R  A  R  Z
B  T  G  O  F  P  A  V  L  Y
E  C  H  E  R  R  I  E  S  V
M  A  E  R  C  E  C  I  T  Z
```

Answers: cheese, chips, chocolate, curry, ice cream, steak. Soporific foods: almonds, oatmeal, cherries, kiwis

Deciding what not to do is as important as deciding what to do.

Steve Jobs

Tonight I decided not to eat _____ right before going to bed.

DATE: __/__/__

Distrust yourself, and sleep well before you fight.

Dr. John Armstrong

I slept well before this "fight":

_____

_____

_____

_____

☐ won ☐ lost ☐ compromised

Night is the wonderful opportunity to take rest, to forgive, to smile, to get ready for all the battles that you have to fight tomorrow.

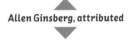

Allen Ginsberg, attributed

Last night I rested, forgave, smiled, and got ready for today's battles:

_____

_____

_____

_____

_____

EACH MORNING SEES
SOME TASK BEGIN,
EACH EVENING SEES
IT CLOSE;
SOMETHING ATTEMPTED,
SOMETHING DONE,
HAS EARNED
A NIGHT'S REPOSE.

Henry Wadsworth Longfellow

DATE: ___/___/___

YESTERDAY'S PROFESSIONAL ACCOMPLISHMENT THAT EARNED ME A NIGHT'S REPOSE:

_____

_____

_____

_____

_____

_____

DATE: ___/___/___

YESTERDAY'S PERSONAL ACCOMPLISHMENT THAT EARNED ME A NIGHT'S REPOSE:

_____

_____

_____

_____

_____

_____

The blues is like this. You lay down some night and you turn from one side of the bed to the other: all night long. It's not too cold in that bed, and it ain't too hot. But what's the matter? The blues has got you.

Leadbelly

The blues that got me last night:

_____

_____

_____

_____

_____

DATE: __/__/__

Me: Please let me sleep!
Brain: Nope, we have to stay up together and go over every bad life decision we have made so far.

Anonymous

Me (last night): Nah, instead let's go over every good life decision, starting with this one:

_____

_____

_____

Rate sleep in Z's: Z Z Z Z

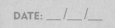
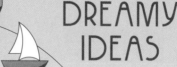

DREAMY IDEAS

Stand Up to Tech

Executives discovered long ago that stand-up
meetings last a significantly shorter time than sit-
downs. This is an insight you can take to bed with you.
If you absolutely need to use an electronic device
when you should be going to sleep, remain standing
the whole time—and *do not* take it to bed with you.
(You probably won't last more than 10 minutes.)

Standing, I logged in at ___:___ P.M.

Standing, I logged out at ___:___ P.M.

How I felt when I got into bed:

_____

Some people can't sleep because they have insomnia. I can't sleep because I have internet.

Anonymous

Before bedtime I did both of these to fight internet insomnia:

☐ silenced my devices

☐ stashed my devices out of reach

Rate sleep in Z's: **Z Z Z Z Z**

I put a piece of paper and a pencil under my pillow, and when I could not sleep, I wrote in the dark.

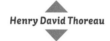

Henry David Thoreau

Something I created when I could not sleep:

_____

_____

_____

_____

_____

Song writing is about getting the demon out of me. It's like being possessed. You try to go to sleep, but the song won't let you. So you have to get up and make it into something, and then you're allowed to sleep.

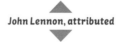

John Lennon, attributed

How the creative process interrupted my sleep:

_____

_____

_____

_____

_____

DATE: __ / __ / __

IN MY DREAM LAST NIGHT I WAS _____.

age

DATE: __ / __ / __

IN MY DREAM LAST NIGHT I WAS _____.

weight

In a dream
you are
never eighty.

Anne Sexton

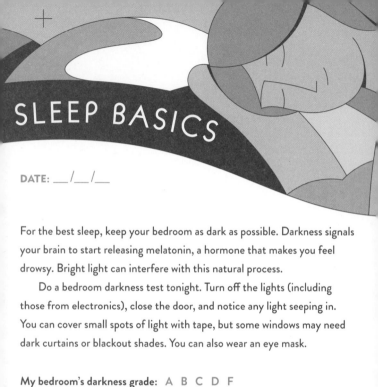

SLEEP BASICS

DATE: ___ / ___ / ___

For the best sleep, keep your bedroom as dark as possible. Darkness signals your brain to start releasing melatonin, a hormone that makes you feel drowsy. Bright light can interfere with this natural process.

Do a bedroom darkness test tonight. Turn off the lights (including those from electronics), close the door, and notice any light seeping in. You can cover small spots of light with tape, but some windows may need dark curtains or blackout shades. You can also wear an eye mask.

My bedroom's darkness grade: A B C D F

My fixes:

_____

_____

_____

_____

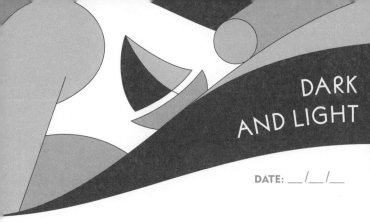

DARK AND LIGHT

Exposure to sunlight during the day, especially in the morning, can actually improve sleep at night by shutting down the release of melatonin. Try to get at least 15 minutes of sunlight first thing in the morning, signaling your brain to wake up. The natural light you get by sitting by a window or going outside on even a gray day can give you four to five times as much light as artificial lighting.

Yesterday I got my 15 minutes of sunlight from ___:___ to ___:___.

Mark how much time you spent outdoors:

Rate sleep in Z's: Z Z Z Z

DATE: ___ / ___ / ___

I love every second of the backbreaking, laborious eighteen-hour days. I have never been so exhausted in my life, and it's perfect. It means I sleep.

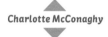

Charlotte McConaghy

My backbreaking day:

_____

_____

_____

_____

Rate sleep in Z's: Z Z Z Z Z

DATE: __/__/__

SWEET IS THE SLEEP OF THE LABORER.

The Bible

☐ My physical labor yesterday:

_____

☐ My mental labor yesterday:

_____

Rate sleep in Z's: Z Z Z Z Z

DATE: ___/___/___

Sleepy *Readings*

Reading for interest should be done
outside the bedroom. Certain texts,
however, can actually be soporific.

What I tried to read last night that put me to sleep:

☐ *Critical and Miscellaneous Essays* by Thomas Carlyle

☐ *Finnegans Wake* by James Joyce

☐ installation instructions for an electronic device

☐ the dictionary

☐ IRS income tax form

☐ _____
　　　　　　　　　other

Rate sleep in Z's: Z Z Z Z Z

The thing to do [for insomnia] is to get an opera score and read that. That will bore you to death.

Marilyn Horne

Last night reading this bored me to death:

_____

_____

_____

_____

_____

THE WOODS ARE LOVELY,
DARK, AND DEEP,
BUT I HAVE PROMISES
TO KEEP,
AND MILES TO GO
BEFORE I SLEEP,
AND MILES TO GO
BEFORE I SLEEP.

Robert Frost

DATE: __ / __ / __

WHAT I PROMISED TO DO TODAY BUT LEFT UNDONE:

_____

_____

_____

_____

_____

_____

DATE: __ / __ / __

HOW I WILL HANDLE TODAY'S UNFULFILLED PROMISES AFTER A REFRESHING NIGHT'S SLEEP:

_____

_____

_____

_____

_____

_____

DATE: ___ / ___ / ___

Come to the woods, for here is rest. There is no repose like that of the green deep woods. Here grow the wallflower and the violet. The squirrel will come and sit upon your knee, the logcock will wake you in the morning. Sleep in forgetfulness of all ill.

John Muir

I sleep best in the country because:

_____

_____

_____

_____

_____

DATE: __ / __ / __

I want to wake up in a city that never sleeps.

Fred Ebb

I sleep best in the city because:

_____

_____

_____

_____

_____

DATE: __/__/__

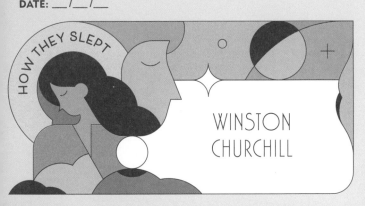

HOW THEY SLEPT

WINSTON CHURCHILL

The British prime minister Winston Churchill slept in segments, a technique called polyphasic sleeping. At 5:00 P.M. Churchill would have a whiskey and take a 2-hour nap. Then he would get up and work until 3:00 A.M. Then to bed for 5 hours and up at 8:00 A.M. Because of this schedule, he often took meetings in his bath.

Last night I tried Churchill's sleep schedule:

_____

_____

_____

Rate sleep in Z's: Z Z Z Z Z

You must sleep some time between lunch and dinner, and no half measures. Take off your clothes and get into bed. Don't think you'll be doing less work. That's a foolish notion held by people who have no imagination.

Winston Churchill

I get ☐ more ☐ less work done when I take a midday nap.

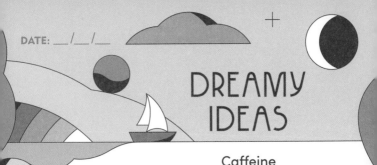

DREAMY IDEAS

Caffeine

Cut off caffeine after 2:00 P.M. Caffeine is a stimulant with a half-life of about 6 to 8 hours and a quarter-life of about 12 hours. You want to clear most of it from your system by the time you go to sleep.

☐ **Did it!**

Rate sleep in Z's: Z Z Z Z Z

Free yourselves from the slavery of the tea and coffee and other slop-kettle.

William Cobbett

My uncaffeinated afternoon drink today:

_____

_____

_____

_____

_____

DATE: ___ / ___ / ___

TODAY I USED MY SUPERPOWER TO:

_____

_____

_____

_____

_____

_____

DATE: ___ / ___ / ___

WITHOUT MY SUPERPOWER I COULDN'T DO THIS TODAY:

_____

_____

_____

_____

_____

_____

Sleep is your superpower.

Matthew Walker

Something nameless Hums us into sleep.

Mark Strand

The nameless thing that hummed me into sleep last night:

_____

_____

_____

_____

_____

Goodnight stars, goodnight air, goodnight noises everywhere.

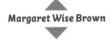

Margaret Wise Brown

Goodnight _____,

goodnight _____,

goodnight _____.

Snoring

Circle the correct answer:

1. Weight <u>gain</u>/<u>loss</u> can make snoring worse.

2. Sleeping on your <u>back</u>/<u>side</u> can reduce snoring.

3. Alcohol <u>increases</u>/<u>decreases</u> your snoring.

4. Muscle relaxants <u>increase</u>/<u>decrease</u> your snoring.

5. Loud and frequent snoring <u>can</u>/<u>cannot</u> be a sign of obstructive sleep apnea.

There ain't no way to find out why a snorer can't hear himself snore.

Mark Twain

Last night I dreamt I went to Manderley again.

Daphne du Maurier

Last night I dreamt I went to _____ again.

I dreamt that I dwelt in marble halls,
With vassals and serfs at my side.

Alfred Bunn

Last night I dreamt that I dwelt in _____.

LYING IN BED JUST BEFORE
GOING TO SLEEP IS THE
WORST TIME FOR *ORGANIZED*
THINKING; IT IS THE BEST TIME
FOR FREE THINKING. IDEAS DRIFT
LIKE CLOUDS IN AN UNDECIDED
BREEZE, TAKING FIRST THIS
DIRECTION AND THEN THAT.

E. L. Konigsburg

DATE: ___ / ___ / ___

A FREE THOUGHT I HAD LAST NIGHT:

_____

_____

_____

_____

_____

_____

DATE: ___ / ___ / ___ .

AN IDEA THAT LED ME IN A NEW DIRECTION LAST NIGHT:

_____

_____

_____

_____

_____

_____

DATE: __/__/__

FATIGUE MAKES COWARDS OF US ALL.

George S. Patton Jr.

I got too little sleep last night and then was afraid to tackle this problem:

_____

_____

_____

☐ Tonight I will sleep my full _____ hours.

DATE: __ / __ / __

When we are tired, we are attacked by ideas we conquered long ago.

Friedrich Nietzsche

I got too little sleep last night and was attacked by these old anxieties:

_____

_____

_____

☐ Tonight I will sleep my full _____ hours.

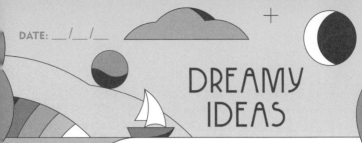

DREAMY IDEAS

Stay Cool in Warm Socks

Is that a mistake, you might ask? No, warming your feet will bring heat to your extremities, cooling off the rest of your body. Wear socks made of breathable materials, such as cotton or wool.

☐ Did it!

Rate sleep in Z's: Z Z Z Z Z

I'm obsessed with socks. I even wear them to bed!

Odette Annable

Draw your favorite sleep socks:

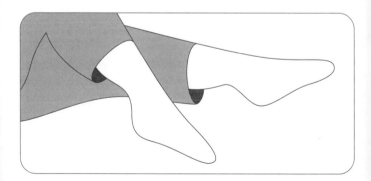

Whoever thinks of going to bed before twelve o'clock is a scoundrel.

Samuel Johnson

Whoever thinks of going to bed after twelve o'clock is _____

_____.

DATE: __ / __ / __

As I grow older I am more and more inclined to believe that night was made for sleep.

Kate Chopin

As I grow older I am more and more inclined to believe _____

_____.

WHAT A REGRET THAT THIS WAS ONLY A DREAM!

_____

_____

_____

_____

_____

_____

WHAT A RELIEF THAT THIS WAS ONLY A DREAM!

_____

_____

_____

_____

_____

_____

So I awoke,
and behold
it was
a dream.

John Bunyan

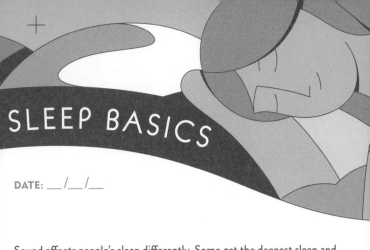

SLEEP BASICS

DATE: __ / __ / __

Sound affects people's sleep differently. Some get the deepest sleep and are less likely to wake up in the night if the bedroom is completely silent. Others find that earplugs or noise-canceling headphones make them too aware of internal body sounds, such as a growling stomach. Many people sleep best with a boring, continuous muffling sound—highway traffic far away from a tall apartment building, a whirring fan, or a white-noise machine or phone app.

Try to control the sudden environmental noises most likely to wake you by either fixing them or muffling them.

Environmental noises I will fix:

☐ creaky floor   ☐ clanking radiator

☐ flapping shade/shutter   ☐ _____
                                          other

☐ squeaky bed

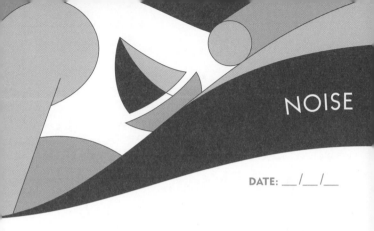

NOISE

DATE: __ / __ / __

Environmental noises I need to muffle:

- ☐ sirens

- ☐ motorcycles

- ☐ howling animals

- ☐ noisy birds or rooster

- ☐ snoring bedmate

- ☐ _____
  other

If they [young software programmers] want we will give them a sleeping bag, but there is something romantic about sleeping under the desk. They want to do it.

Bill Gates

I have slept: ☐ under a desk

☐ under the stars

☐ under a bunk bed

☐ under a tent

☐ under a _____
other

I sometimes doubt that a writer should refine or improve his workroom by so much as a dictionary: one thing leads to another and the first thing you know he has a stuffed chair and is fast asleep in it.

E. B. White

Where I napped today:

_____

_____

_____

_____

_____

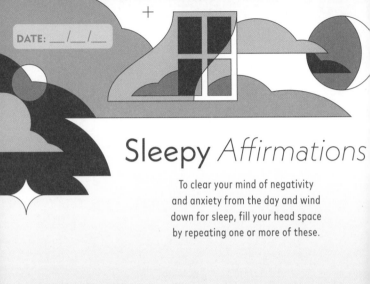

DATE: __ / __ / __

Sleepy *Affirmations*

To clear your mind of negativity
and anxiety from the day and wind
down for sleep, fill your head space
by repeating one or more of these.

Last night I told myself:

☐ I've done my best today.

☐ I am grateful for all my life's experiences.

☐ I let go of fear, worry, and anger, and I welcome happiness.

☐ I give myself permission to close my eyes and wake refreshed.

☐ Tomorrow is a new day full of possibilities.

☐ _____
other

Rate sleep in Z's: Z Z Z Z Z

Before you fall asleep every day, say something positive to yourself.

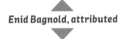

Enid Bagnold, attributed

Something positive I said to myself last night:

_____

_____

_____

_____

_____

THE BEST
ERASER IN
THE WORLD
IS A GOOD
NIGHT'S SLEEP.

Orlando A. Battista

DATE: ___/___/___

A WORRY ERASED BY LAST NIGHT'S SLEEP:

_____

_____

_____

_____

_____

_____

DATE: ___/___/___

AN EMBARRASSMENT ERASED BY LAST NIGHT'S SLEEP:

_____

_____

_____

_____

_____

DATE: ___ / ___ / ___

I had a poem in my head last night, flashing as only those unformed midnight poems can. It was all made up of unexpected burning words. . . . Now not a word of it remains, not even a hint of its direction. What a pity one cannot sleepwrite on the ceiling with one's finger or lifted toe.

Denton Welch

I had a flash of inspiration last night for a ☐ poem ☐ song ☐ screenplay ☐ painting ☐ _____.

other

(It was brilliant, unique, awesome—if only I could remember it.)

I get up in the morning with an idea for a three-volume novel and by nightfall it's a paragraph in my column.

Don Marquis

The A+ idea I had on awakening:

_____

_____

_____

Grade by nightfall: _____

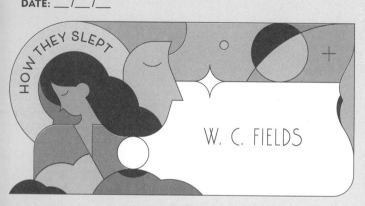

HOW THEY SLEPT

W. C. FIELDS

Comedian W. C. Fields was an insomniac who couldn't sleep unless it was raining. To solve this problem, he put a sprinkler under an umbrella to mimic the noise.

For me, the ideal weather for sleeping is:

_____

_____

_____

_____

_____

The best cure for insomnia is to get a lot of sleep.

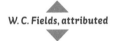

W. C. Fields, attributed

For me, the best cure for insomnia is:

_____

_____

_____

_____

_____

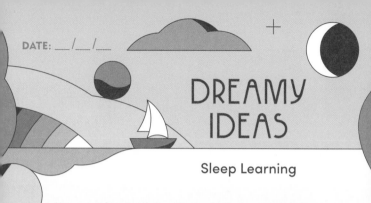

DREAMY IDEAS

Sleep Learning

Use your sleeping hours strategically to consolidate information you studied that day. Deep sleep is the best time for learning facts, such as names, dates, or vocabulary. To get the most deep sleep, which occurs in the first part of the night, go to bed at your regular time and do a quick review when you wake up.

Last night I prepared for _____ **by:**

_____

_____

_____

It ☐ did ☐ did not work.

DATE: __ / __ / __

I think of sleep as learning with my eyes closed.

Benedict Carey

What I learned in my sleep last night:

_____

_____

_____

_____

_____

DATE: __ / __ / __

TEST I PASSED TODAY IN SPITE OF BEING SOOOO TIRED:

_____

_____

_____

_____

_____

_____

DATE: __ / __ / __

TEST I FAILED TODAY BECAUSE I WAS SOOOO TIRED:

_____

_____

_____

_____

_____

_____

The test
of a people
is what
they can do
when they're
tired.

Winston Churchill

I never take a nap after dinner but when I have had a bad night, and then the nap takes me.

Samuel Johnson

Why a nap took me today:

_____

_____

_____

_____

_____

It's been a hard day's night.
I should be sleeping like a log.

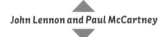

John Lennon and Paul McCartney

It was a hard day's night. I slept like a _____.

QUIZ 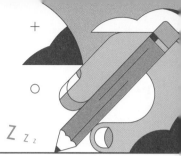 Z Z z z z

Winding Down for a Perfect Night's Sleep

Write your ideal bedtime here: _____

Now mark the times on the clocks below when you should stop the corresponding activities:

a. drinking coffee

d. exercising

b. drinking alcohol

e. working

c. eating dinner

f. using electronic devices

Answers: a. 4 hours before bedtime; b. 3 hours before bedtime; c. 2 to 3 hours before bedtime; d. 2 hours before bedtime; e. and f. 1 hour before bedtime

DATE: ___/___/___

The final test of a plan is its execution.

U.S. Army

☐ I executed the recommended winding-down plan.

Rate sleep in Z's: Z Z Z Z Z

Bed is the poor man's opera.

Italian proverb

For me, bed is my front-row seat at _____.

(My) definition of luxury is sleep, sleep, sleep, sleep. Just a great bed and sleeping.

Tom Ford

Why sleep is a luxury for me:

_____

_____

_____

_____

_____

I'VE DREAMT IN MY LIFE
DREAMS THAT HAVE STAYED
WITH ME EVER AFTER, AND
CHANGED MY IDEAS: THEY'VE
GONE THROUGH AND
THROUGH ME, LIKE WINE
THROUGH WATER, AND ALTERED
THE COLOR OF MY MIND.

Emily Brontë

DATE: ___ / ___ / ___

A DREAM THAT CHANGED AN IDEA LAST NIGHT:

_____

_____

_____

_____

_____

_____

DATE: ___ / ___ / ___

A DREAM THAT ALTERED THE COLOR OF MY MIND LAST NIGHT:

_____

_____

_____

_____

_____

_____

DATE: __/__/__

I come to the office each morning and stay for long hours doing what has to be done to the best of my ability. And when you've done the best you can, you can't do any better. So when I go to sleep I turn everything over to the Lord and forget it.

Harry S. Truman

☐ Yesterday I did my work to the best of my ability.

☐ Then I let it go and went to sleep.

Rate sleep in Z's: **Z Z Z Z Z**

I believe the greatest asset a head of state can have is the ability to get a good night's sleep.

Harold Wilson

☐ I was a leader at work today after last night's good sleep:

_____

_____

_____

_____

_____

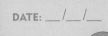

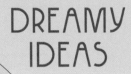

DREAMY IDEAS

Bed = Sleep and Sex Only

Most experts recommend restricting the bed to only two activities: sleep and sex. Being strict and consistent is the only way to train your subconscious brain to expect this. If you do other activities in bed (even reading), you weaken the association, which should be working in your favor when it is time to go to sleep.

I ☐ do ☐ do not need to strengthen my brain's sleepy-time associations with my bed.

If possible, you should always sleep with someone you love. You both recharge your mutual batteries free of charge.

Marlene Dietrich

Last night I slept with someone I love:

_____

_____

How I feel:

_____

_____

He dreamed he was eating shredded wheat and woke up to find the mattress half gone.

Fred Allen

Sign of my restless sleep last night:

_____

_____

_____

_____

_____

DATE: __ / __ / __

Last night I dreamed I ate a ten-pound marshmallow, and when I woke up, the pillow was gone.

Tommy Cooper

Sign of my wild dream last night:

_____

_____

_____

_____

_____

DATE: ___ / ___ / ___

SLEEP PHOBIA #1:

_____

_____

_____

_____

_____

_____

DATE: ___ / ___ / ___

SLEEP PHOBIA #2:

_____

_____

_____

_____

_____

_____

I have three phobias which, could I mute them, would make my life as slick as a sonnet, but as dull as ditch water: I hate to go to bed, I hate to get up, and I hate to be alone.

Tallulah Bankhead

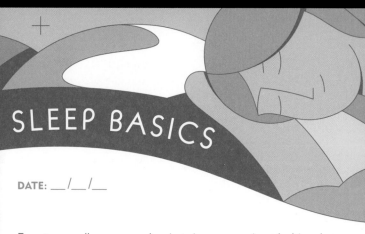

SLEEP BASICS

DATE: __ / __ / __

Experts generally recommend against vigorous exercise at bedtime, but most are in favor of stretching and meditative movements like yoga as a calming transition to sleep. Try one of these yoga poses tonight.

☐ <u>Child's pose</u> releases tension in the back and shoulders and stretches the hips. Get on your hands and knees and slowly lower your butt toward your heels. Hold this position for 30 seconds. Repeat three times.

☐ <u>Legs-up-the-wall pose</u> reduces swelling in the legs. Lie on the floor close to a wall, and lift your legs, resting them on the wall. Hold this pose for 1 to 2 minutes.

Rate sleep in Z's: Z Z Z Z Z

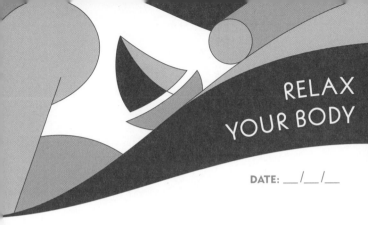

Here are two soothing stretches to try in bed.

☐ <u>**Full-body stretch**</u>. Extend your right arm straight up, reaching as high as you can toward the ceiling, until you feel your whole right side stretch. Repeat with your left arm.

☐ <u>**Back stretch**</u>. Lie flat on your back in bed. Push your spine into the bed, flattening your back and pulling in your abdomen. Release all your muscles, and breathe deeply. Repeat this several times until you are lying limp.

Rate sleep in Z's: Z Z Z Z Z

DATE: __ / __ / __

Marriage is an alliance entered into
by a man who can't sleep with the
window shut, and a woman who
can't sleep with the window open.

George Bernard Shaw, attributed

Accommodation I ☐ make ☐ would make for a sleep partner:

_____

_____

_____

_____

_____

DATE: ___/___/___

I'll have to have a room of my own.
Nobody could sleep with Dick. He
wakes up during the night, switches
on the lights, and speaks into his tape
recorder or takes notes.

Pat Nixon

Accommodation I ☐ don't make ☐ would not make for a sleep

partner:

_____

_____

_____

_____

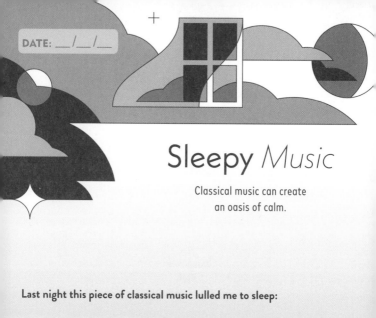

DATE: __ / __ / __

Sleepy *Music*

Classical music can create
an oasis of calm.

Last night this piece of classical music lulled me to sleep:

☐ Frédéric Chopin's Nocturne in E-flat Major, op. 9, no. 2

☐ Maurice Ravel's Piano Concerto in G Major, 2nd movement

☐ Ludwig van Beethoven's "Moonlight" Sonata, 1st movement

☐ J. S. Bach's Prelude no. 1 in C Major

☐ W. A. Mozart's Flute and Harp Concerto, 2nd movement

☐ _____
  other

Rate sleep in Z's: Z Z Z Z Z

DATE: __ / __ / __

Music hath charms to soothe a savage breast,
To soften rocks, or bend a knotted oak.

William Congreve

A melody that charmed me to sleep:

_____

_____

_____

_____

_____

PEOPLE DON'T
REALIZE HOW
IMPORTANT IT
IS TO WAKE UP
EVERY MORNING
WITH A SONG IN
YOUR HEART.

Jiddu Krishnamurti, attributed

DATE: ___ / ___ / ___

THE SONG IN MY HEART THIS MORNING:

☐ "Oh, What a Beautiful Mornin'"

☐ _____
                        other

DATE: ___ / ___ / ___

THE SONG IN MY HEART THIS MORNING:

☐ "Oh! How I Hate to Get Up in the Morning"

☐ _____
                        other

DATE: ___ /___ /___

It is comforting when one has a sorrow to lie in the warmth of one's bed and there, abandoning all effort and all resistance, to bury even one's head under the cover, giving one's self up to it completely, moaning like branches in the autumn wind.

Marcel Proust

How my bed was a comfort last night:

_____

_____

_____

_____

_____

DATE: __ / __ / __

There have been times in my life when I have
fallen asleep in tears; but in my dreams the
most charming forms have come to console
and to cheer me, and I have risen the next
morning fresh and joyful.

Johann Wolfgang von Goethe

How my dreams cheered me last night:

_____

_____

_____

_____

_____

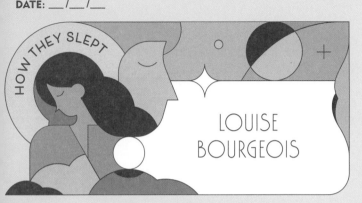

HOW THEY SLEPT

LOUISE BOURGEOIS

Artist Louise Bourgeois suffered from bouts of insomnia throughout her life, but she dealt with them by using her sleeplessness to create works of art. Her *Insomnia Drawings* contains drawings, sketches, and poetic annotations.

My insomniac artwork from last night:

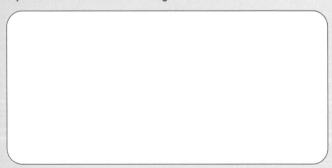

Lying in bed would be an altogether perfect and supreme experience if only one had a colored pencil long enough to draw on the ceiling.

G. K. Chesterton

Lying in bed would be an altogether perfect and supreme experience if only:

_____

_____

_____

_____

_____

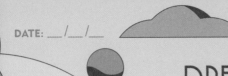

DREAMY IDEAS

Countdown to Sleep

Counting sheep is a popular but unproven strategy for falling asleep. Some researchers believe that the key is to choose a theme that requires just the right amount of mental energy to provide distraction from anxious thoughts but not to itself cause stress. This may be reciting and visualizing the stops on a long train commute; American states or countries of the world; stars in the Western Hemisphere; names of players on football or soccer teams.

What I counted last night to put myself to sleep:

_____

Rate sleep in Z's: Z Z Z Z Z

DATE: ___/___/___

[Sleep] covers a man all over, thoughts and all, like a cloak; 'tis meat for the hungry, drink for the thirsty, heat for the cold, and cold for the hot.

Miguel de Cervantes

To me, sleep is:

_____

_____

_____

_____

_____

DATE: __/__/__

TODAY I SLEPT INSTEAD OF:

_____

_____

_____

_____

_____

_____

DATE: __/__/__

TODAY I DOZED OFF DURING:

_____

_____

_____

_____

_____

_____

Never waste any time you can spend sleeping.

Frank Knight

I have no trouble with my enemies. I can take care of my enemies all right. But my damn friends. . . . They're the ones that keep me walking the floor nights!

Warren G. Harding

A worry about a friend that kept me walking the floor last night:

_____

_____

_____

_____

_____

DATE: __/__/__

Great events make me quiet and calm; it is only trifles that irritate my nerves.

Queen Victoria

A trifle that irritated my nerves last night:

_____

_____

_____

_____

_____

DATE: __ / __ / __

QUIZ z z z z

Make This Bedroom Ready for Sleep

Draw what you need in this bedroom to sleep well.

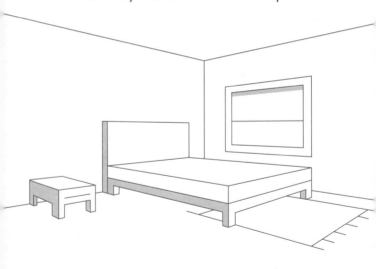

Answers: Must include blinds, pillow, blanket, and thermostat set at 65°F; must not have clock or any electronic devices.

REAL COMFORT, VISUAL AND PHYSICAL, IS VITAL TO EVERY ROOM.

Mark Hampton

Comforting visual element in my bedroom:

_____

Comforting physical element in my bedroom:

_____

They could see she was a real Princess and no question about it, now that she had felt one pea all the way through twenty mattresses and twenty more feather beds. Nobody but a Princess could be so delicate.

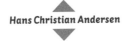

Hans Christian Andersen

Bedding requirements that prove I am royalty:

_____

_____

_____

_____

_____

My mother gets all mad at me if I stay in a hotel. I'm 31 years old, and I don't want to sleep on a sleeping bag down in the basement.

Ben Affleck

Most uncomfortable place I had to sleep to keep peace in the family:

_____

_____

_____

_____

_____

KNOWING YOU HAVE
SOMETHING GOOD
TO READ BEFORE
BED IS AMONG THE
MOST PLEASURABLE
OF SENSATIONS.

Vladimir Nabokov

DATE: __ / __ / __

FICTION I LOOK FORWARD TO READING TONIGHT BEFORE BED:

_____

_____

_____

_____

.

_____

_____

DATE: __ / __ / __

NONFICTION I LOOK FORWARD TO READING TONIGHT BEFORE BED:

_____

_____

_____

_____

_____

_____

DATE: __ / __ / __

The greatest weariness comes from work not done.

Eric Hoffer

☐ I finished my work before going to bed.

Rate sleep in Z's: Z Z Z Z Z

I have so much to do that I am going to bed.

Savoyard proverb

☐ I didn't finish my work before going to bed.

Rate sleep in Z's: **Z Z Z Z Z**

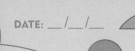

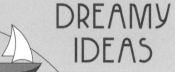

DREAMY IDEAS

Sleeping with Pets

Pet owners have traditionally been discouraged from sleeping with their pets. Animals can trigger allergies, introduce germs, and disrupt sleep with their noises and movements. Yet about half of cat and dog owners ignore this advice. Studies have also shown that, for some people, sleeping with pets provides comfort and a sense of security. So if you have a pet, you have to decide for yourself.

My position on sleeping with a pet:

_____

_____

_____

Collapsing into bed [after a night of dancing in cabarets], I would snuggle against my puppies and sleep until the maid awakened me at four.

Josephine Baker

Who or what I snuggled with last night:

_____

_____

_____

Rate sleep in Z's: Z Z Z Z Z

I can neither eat nor sleep for thinking of you my dearest love.

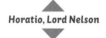

Horatio, Lord Nelson

Last night I could not sleep for thinking of _____.

I don't mind sleeping on an empty stomach provided it isn't my own.

Philip J. Simborg

My favorite empty stomach to sleep on:

_____

_____

_____

_____

_____

DATE: ___ / ___ / ___

DREAM LAST NIGHT WITH TEARS AND TORTURE:

_____

_____

_____

_____

_____

_____

DATE: ___ / ___ / ___

DREAM LAST NIGHT WITH BREATH AND THE TOUCH OF JOY:

_____

_____

_____

_____

_____

SLEEP HATH ITS
OWN WORLD,
AND A WIDE REALM
OF WILD REALITY.
AND DREAMS IN THEIR
DEVELOPMENT HAVE BREATH,
AND TEARS, AND TORTURES,
AND THE TOUCH OF JOY.

Lord Byron

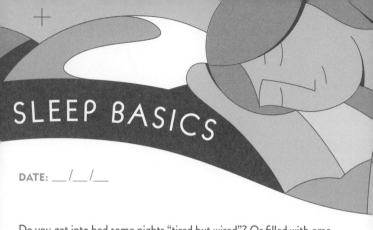

SLEEP BASICS

DATE: __ / __ / __

Do you get into bed some nights "tired but wired"? Or filled with emotional stress? If so, these practices, rooted in Eastern religion, may soothe your mind. Check a new one that you will try tonight or tried last night.

☐ <u>Breathing</u>: Take deep, slow breaths after you lie down. If your mind is racing, this should slow it down as it slows your heart rate.

☐ <u>Mantra</u>: Close your eyes and recite a calming word or short phrase— "sleep," "let it go," or the Hindu "om."

☐ <u>Meditation</u>: This involves focusing on an experience in the here and now—a birdsong, even your own breath. You can do this on your own or use a meditation app.

Rate sleep in Z's: Z Z Z Z Z

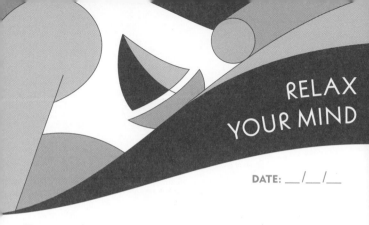

These mental relaxation practices have more eclectic origins. They are meant to redirect your mind from stress to calm. Check a new one that you will try tonight or tried last night.

☐ <u>Gratitude</u>. For some people, counting their blessings rather than sheep sets the mind in a positive direction.

☐ <u>Affirmation</u>. Finding a positive statement to repeat to yourself can offset your worries. "I am effective"; "I am loved."

☐ <u>Visualization</u>. Call up a picture in your mind of a generic beautiful, relaxing scene in nature or a personal one filled with fond memories.

☐ <u>Writing</u>. Keep a worry journal by your bed and spill your anxieties into it before you go to sleep.

Rate sleep in Z's: Z Z Z Z Z

DATE: __ / __ / __

To rise at six, to dine at ten,
To sup at six, to sleep at ten,
Makes a man live for ten
times ten.

Victor Hugo

My schedule: To rise at _____, to dine at _____,

To sup at _____, to sleep at _____.

So far, I have lived for _____.

The slightest interruption in the household routine completely de-rails me.

Edith Wharton

Yesterday's interruption in the household schedule that completely de-railed my sleep last night:

_____

_____

_____

_____

_____

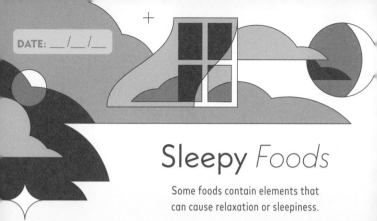

DATE: ___ / ___ / ___

Sleepy *Foods*

Some foods contain elements that
can cause relaxation or sleepiness.

To help me sleep last night, I ate:

☐ cherries, with melatonin, to help control my sleep/wake cycle

☐ bread, with carbohydrates, for energy and then a crash

☐ almonds, a source of melatonin

☐ turkey, high in tryptophan, to promote sleep quality

☐ bananas, with potassium and magnesium, to help relax
my muscles

☐ _____
other

Rate sleep in Z's: Z Z Z Z Z

DATE: __ / __ / __

It is said that the effect of eating too much lettuce is "soporific."

Beatrix Potter

I can say from last night's experience that eating too much

_____ is soporific.

NIGHT IS THE MOTHER OF THOUGHTS.

John Florio

DATE: __ / __ / __

BRILLIANT THOUGHT I HAD LAST NIGHT:

_____

_____

_____

_____

_____

_____

DATE: __ / __ / __

NOT-SO-BRILLIANT THOUGHT I HAD LAST NIGHT:

_____

_____

_____

_____

_____

_____

DATE: __ / __ / __

He that sleeps feels not the tooth-ache.

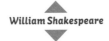

William Shakespeare

Physical pain that disappeared as I slept last night:

_____

_____

_____

_____

_____

O magic sleep! O comfortable bird,
That broodest o'er the troubled sea
   of mind
Till it is hush'd and smooth!

John Keats

Emotional pain that disappeared as I slept last night:

_____

_____

_____

_____

_____

DATE: __ / __ / __

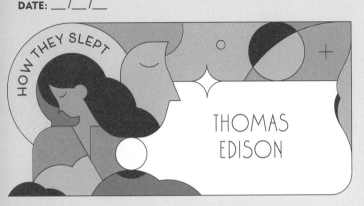

HOW THEY SLEPT

THOMAS EDISON

Inventor Thomas Edison owed his success "to the fact that I never had a clock in my workroom. Seventy-five of us worked twenty hours every day and slept only four hours—and thrived on it."

The least amount of sleep I can get and thrive the next day: _____

Last night I had only _____ hours of sleep and today I am

☐ thriving ☐ a mess ☐ _____
                                                        other

Happiness consists in getting enough sleep. Just that, nothing more.

Robert A. Heinlein

Enough sleep for me, nothing more: _____

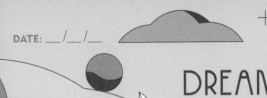

DREAMY IDEAS

Jet Lag Trick

Jet lag occurs when you knock your internal clock off kilter by flying across time zones. You feel tired during the day (nighttime at home) and are unable to fall asleep or stay asleep at night (daytime at home). The bigger the time change, the longer this lasts. To help prevent jet lag, start several days before your trip shifting the times you sleep and eat meals an hour closer to those of your destination. Then, when you land, adopt the local clock completely.

I ☐ tried   ☐ will try this trick.

It ☐ worked   ☐ did not work for me.

I shall sleep, and move with the moving ships,
Change as the winds change, veer in the tide.

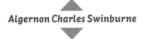

Algernon Charles Swinburne

Why is it harder to "change as the winds change" flying east than flying west?

☐ 1. The sun shines brighter in the east.

☐ 2. The air is drier in the west.

☐ 3. It is easier to stay up late than go to bed early.

Answers: It is true that sunlight affects your internal clock and that dehydration can increase symptoms of jet lag, but answer 3 is correct.

DATE: __ / __ / __

WHAT GOT ME OUT OF BED IN A GOOD MOOD THIS MORNING:

- ☐ birds chirping
- ☐ coffee brewing
- ☐ sunlight
- ☐ kisses
- ☐ _____
  other

DATE: __ / __ / __

WHAT GOT ME OUT OF BED IN A BAD MOOD THIS MORNING:

- ☐ sirens
- ☐ work intrusion
- ☐ loud voices
- ☐ bad weather
- ☐ _____
  other

He has his law degree and a furnished office. It's just a question of getting him out of bed.

Peter Arno

DATE: __/__/__

I can tell you with authority that when I'm exhausted, when I'm running on empty, I'm the worst version of myself. I'm more reactive. I'm less empathetic. I'm less creative.

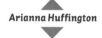

Arianna Huffington

I was so exhausted today from too little sleep that I was more

_____ and less _____.

I got so involved in the urgency of the situation [pandemic] that I was not sleeping more than 4 hours a night. . . . It really took my wife to shake me and say, "Hey, you know this is going to be a marathon. . . . If you think you're in a sprint, you're going to burn out fast."

Anthony Fauci

☐ Yesterday I didn't allow a crisis to interrupt my full night's sleep, so this morning I will be able to handle it.

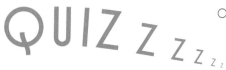
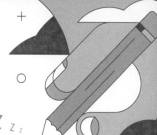

QUIZ ZZ z z z

Bedtime Checklist

Fill in the blanks with what you should do before going to bed.

1. Write a list of what you are _____ for.

2. Make the room as _____, _____,

   and _____ as possible.

3. No cup of _____ after 2:00 P.M.

4. Take a _____ bath or shower.

5. Turn off all _____ devices.

When I was young, I started picking out my outfits the night before school, and I still do this! I lay out everything from my underwear to my jewelry. I also pack my backpack and purse. This ritual gives me a sense of tranquility before bedtime.

Amanda Hesser

Ritual that gives me a sense of tranquility before bedtime:

_____

_____

_____

_____

_____

DATE: ___ / ___ / ___

In the long succession of beds in which I spent the nights of my childhood ... the combination of bed and book granted me a sort of home which I knew I could go back to, night after night, under whichever skies.

Alberto Manguel

The combination of bed and _____ was a comfort in my childhood.

DATE: ___/___/___

Another thing I need to do, when I'm near the end of [writing] the book, is sleep in the same room with it. . . . Somehow the book doesn't leave you when you're asleep right next to it.

Joan Didion

Last night I slept better because I kept _____ in my bedroom.

MANY'S THE LONG
NIGHT I'VE DREAMED
OF CHEESE—
TOASTED, MOSTLY.

Robert Louis Stevenson

DATE: ___ / ___ / ___

MANY'S THE LONG NIGHT I'VE DREAMED OF _____.

food

DATE: ___ / ___ / ___

MANY'S THE LONG NIGHT I'VE DREAMED OF _____.

place

More anger stems from lack of sleep than from all of life's frustrations.

D. Sutten

I didn't sleep last night and today blew up at _____.

Without enough sleep, we all become tall two-year-olds.

JoJo Jensen

Tantrum I had today because I didn't get enough sleep:

_____

_____

_____

_____

_____

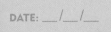

DREAMY IDEAS

Dedicated Sleepwear

Choose bedclothes that your mind will associate only with sleep. No need for silk or satin. An oversized cotton T-shirt is fine, but gym clothes are a big no-no—they send the opposite message.

Draw your coziest dedicated sleepwear:

DATE: __ / __ / __

[Reporters] ask you questions. . . . "What do you wear to bed? Do you wear a pajama top, the bottoms of the pajamas, or a nightgown?" So I said, "Chanel No. 5," because it's the truth.

Marilyn Monroe

What did you wear to bed last night?

_____

_____

_____

_____

_____

Rate sleep in Z's: Z Z Z Z Z

Insomnia is a gross feeder. It will nourish itself on any kind of thinking, including thinking about not thinking.

Clifton Fadiman

I will meditate tonight and stop thinking about this:

_____

_____

_____

_____

_____

DATE: __/__/__

MY EYELIDS ARE HEAVY, BUT MY THOUGHTS ARE HEAVIER.

Unknown

Heavy thoughts I must put aside tonight:

_____

_____

_____

_____

_____

DATE: __ / __ / __

MY POETIC THOUGHT LAST NIGHT:

_____

_____

_____

_____

_____

_____

DATE: __ / __ / __

MY TRUE THOUGHT LAST NIGHT:

_____

_____

_____

_____

_____

_____

POETRY IS . . . THAT
TIME OF NIGHT, LYING
IN BED, THINKING WHAT
YOU REALLY THINK,
MAKING THE PRIVATE
WORLD PUBLIC, THAT'S
WHAT THE POET DOES.

Allen Ginsberg

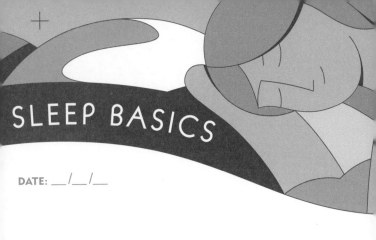

SLEEP BASICS

DATE: __ / __ / __

Sleep experts recommend turning off all screens—TVs, computers, tablets, cell phones—at least 30 to 60 minutes before bedtime and moving all devices out of the bedroom. The blue light they emit can suppress the production of melatonin, the hormone that promotes sleep. If you must occasionally use an electronic device right before bedtime, choose one with a program that reduces blue-light exposure. Even that, though, will not prevent the sleep-thwarting stimulation of reading email or scanning Twitter.

Last night I turned off all my devices at _____.

I went to bed at _____.

Rate sleep in Z's: Z Z Z Z Z

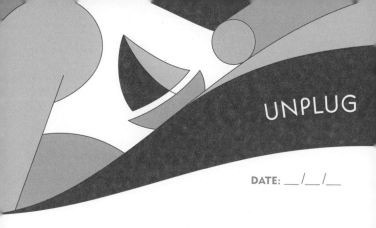

UNPLUG

DATE: ___/___/___

Last night I filled the half hour before my bedtime with these screen-free activities:

☐ listening to soothing music

☐ sketching

☐ reading a book or magazine (print)

☐ knitting

☐ _____
other

Rate sleep in Z's: Z Z Z Z Z

The breeze at dawn has secrets to tell you, Don't go back to sleep.

Rumi

☐ I listened to the breeze this morning.

It was such a lovely day I thought it was a pity to get up.

W. Somerset Maugham

Good weather makes me want to ☐ get up ☐ sleep longer.

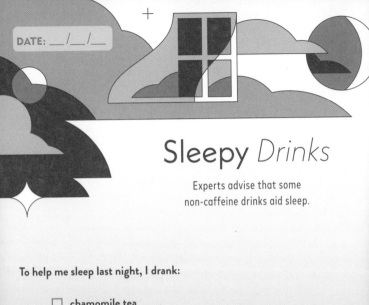

DATE: ___ / ___ / ___

Sleepy *Drinks*

Experts advise that some
non-caffeine drinks aid sleep.

To help me sleep last night, I drank:

- ☐ chamomile tea

- ☐ warm milk

- ☐ cherry juice

- ☐ valerian tea

- ☐ peppermint tea

- ☐ lavender tea

- ☐ _____
  other

Rate sleep in Z's: Z Z Z Z Z

There is a real encounter between me and the tea, and peace, happiness, and joy are possible during the time I drink.

Thich Nhat Hanh

How I felt while I was drinking my sleepy drink last night:

_____

_____

_____

_____

_____

A WELL-SPENT DAY BRINGS HAPPY SLEEP.

Leonardo da Vinci

DATE: __ / __ / __

MY WELL-SPENT YESTERDAY AT WORK:

_____

_____

_____

_____

I ☐ DID   ☐ DID NOT   HAVE A HAPPY SLEEP.

DATE: __ / __ / __

MY WELL-SPENT YESTERDAY WITH FAMILY OR FRIENDS:

_____

_____

_____

_____

I ☐ DID   ☐ DID NOT   HAVE A HAPPY SLEEP.

For sleep, one needs endless depths of blackness to sink into; daylight is too shallow, it will not cover one.

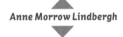

Anne Morrow Lindbergh

How I made my room completely dark last night:

_____

_____

_____

_____

_____

DATE: ___/___/___

I climbed the roofs at break of day;
Sun-smitten Alps before me lay.

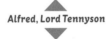

Alfred, Lord Tennyson

Where I got my dose of sunlight this morning:

_____

_____

_____

_____

_____

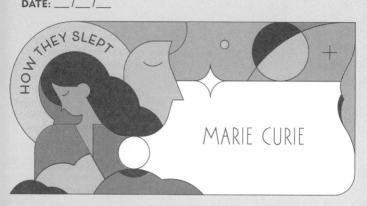

The scientist Marie Curie, who won two Nobel Prizes for her discoveries about radiation, slept with a jar of radium, which she used as a night-light, at her bedside. Unfortunately, the exposure to radium contributed to her death.

Where I leave my work before I go to bed:

_____

_____

_____

_____

_____

I'm not lonely, and I think that has a lot to do with what's on my bedside table rather than what's in my bed.

Michelle Williams

Draw what's on your bedside table.

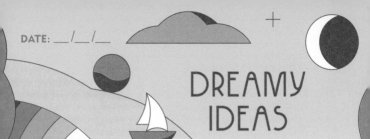

DREAMY IDEAS

Perfect Pillow

The best pillow aligns your head and neck in the same relative position to your spine as when you're standing. Side-sleepers need fluffy pillows. Back- and stomach-sleepers can be comfortable with flatter pillows.

I sleep on my _____.

Draw a picture of your perfect pillow:

Fatigue is the best pillow.

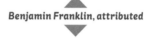

Benjamin Franklin, attributed

For me, _____ is the best pillow.

DATE: ___ / ___ / ___

I DIDN'T LOSE SLEEP OVER THIS PUBLIC PROBLEM:

_____

_____

_____

_____

_____

_____

DATE: ___ / ___ / ___

I DID LOSE SLEEP OVER THIS PERSONAL PROBLEM:

_____

_____

_____

_____

_____

_____

No man should ever lose sleep over public affairs.

Harold Macmillan

DATE: ___/___/___

It seemed to be a necessary ritual that he should prepare himself for sleep by meditating under the solemnity of the night sky.

Victor Hugo

☐ I meditated outdoors before going to bed last night.

Rate sleep in Z's: Z Z Z Z Z

DATE: ___ / ___ / ___

[Meditation] is the power that leads you to your own truth. . . . The main thing meditation frees you from is the idea of "do-ership," the thinking that "I am doing this."

Phylicia Rashad

☐ I meditated, doing nothing, last night as I fell asleep.

Rate sleep in Z's: Z Z Z Z Z

QUIZ Z Z Z z z

Sleep Dictionary

Match up the vocabulary word with its definition.

1. circadian rhythm

2. REM

3. melatonin

4. apnea

5. tryptophan

6. insomnia

a) hormone released by the brain in darkness to help you sleep

b) disorder in falling and/or staying asleep

c) sleep disorder that causes a momentary halt in breathing

d) natural process that regulates the 24-hour sleep/wake cycle

e) stage of sleep when dreaming occurs

f) amino acid found in foods that helps calm and regulate sleep

Answers: 1. d; 2. e; 3. a; 4. c; 5. f; 6. b

DATE: __/__/__

From <u>The Devil's Dictionary</u>:

TZETZE (or TSETSE) FLY, n. An African insect (*Glossina morsitans*) whose bite is commonly regarded as nature's most efficacious remedy for insomnia, though some patients prefer that of the American novelist (*Mendax interminabilis*).

Ambrose Bierce

Bedtime reading that cured my insomnia last night:

_____

_____

_____

_____

_____

Take thou of me, sweet pillowes,
    sweetest bed;
A chamber deafe of noise, and blind
    of light,
A rosie garland and a weary hed.

Sir Philip Sidney

A conventional place I slept last night:

_____

_____

_____

_____

Rate sleep in Z's: Z Z Z Z Z

DATE: __/__/__

Sleeping in a bed—it is, apparently, of immense importance. Against those who sleep, from choice or necessity, elsewhere society feels righteously hostile. It is not done. It is disorderly, anarchical.

Rose Macaulay

An unconventional place I slept last night:

_____

_____

_____

_____

Rate sleep in Z's: Z Z Z Z Z

WHEN YOU DREAM, YOU
DIALOGUE WITH ASPECTS OF
YOURSELF THAT NORMALLY
ARE NOT WITH YOU IN
THE DAYTIME AND YOU
DISCOVER THAT YOU KNOW
A GREAT DEAL MORE THAN
YOU THOUGHT YOU DID.

Toni Cade Bambara

DATE: __ / __ / __

CONVERSATION I HAD WITH MYSELF IN A DREAM LAST NIGHT:

_____

_____

_____

_____

_____

_____

DATE: __ / __ / __

HOW KNOWLEDGEABLE I WAS ABOUT _____ IN MY

DREAM CONVERSATION LAST NIGHT!

DATE: ___ / ___ / ___

I have never taken any exercise,
except sleeping and resting, and
I never intend to take any.

Mark Twain

Number these exercises in order of preference:

_____ swimming

_____ running

_____ tennis

_____ sleeping

_____ basketball

_____ skiing

_____ _____
               other

Star the exercise you did yesterday.

Rate sleep in Z's: **Z Z Z Z Z**

Walk groundly, talk profoundly, drink roundly, sleep soundly.

William Hazlitt

☐ I walked groundly

☐ I talked profoundly

☐ I drank roundly (3 hours before bedtime, of course)

And last night I ☐ did ☐ did not sleep soundly

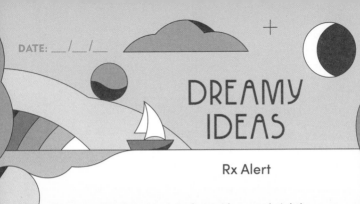

DREAMY IDEAS

Rx Alert

Some medications can interfere with a good night's sleep. These include drugs prescribed for heart disease, blood pressure, or asthma as well as over-the-counter or herbal remedies for coughs, colds, or allergies. Ask your doctor if changing the timing of your medications might improve your sleep.

I will ask my doctor about these medications today:

Medicine	Recommendation

The patient must combat the disease along with the physician.

Hippocrates

I talked to my doctor about my medications and made this change:

_____

_____

_____

_____

_____

Rate sleep in Z's: Z Z Z Z Z

Good night now, and rest. Today was a test. You passed it, you're past it. Now breathe till unstressed.

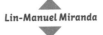

Lin-Manuel Miranda

Whew! I passed this test today:

_____

_____

_____

_____

_____

There are two days in the week
about which and upon which
I never worry. . . . One of these is
Yesterday. . . . And the other day
I do not worry about is Tomorrow.

Robert Jones Burdette

I didn't worry about this last night:

_____

_____

_____

_____

Rate sleep in Z's: Z Z Z Z Z

DATE: ___ / ___ / ___

I WENT TO BED ON SCHEDULE LIKE WHISTLER'S MOTHER. THIS IS HOW I
FELT IN THE MORNING:

_____

_____

_____

_____

_____

DATE: ___ / ___ / ___

I WENT OUT PARTYING AND LEFT WHISTLER'S MOTHER AT HOME. THIS IS
HOW I FELT IN THE MORNING:

_____

_____

_____

_____

_____

The less I behave like Whistler's mother the night before, the more I look like her the morning after.

Tallulah Bankhead

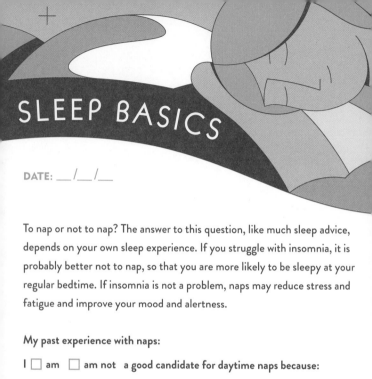

SLEEP BASICS

DATE: __ /__ /__

To nap or not to nap? The answer to this question, like much sleep advice, depends on your own sleep experience. If you struggle with insomnia, it is probably better not to nap, so that you are more likely to be sleepy at your regular bedtime. If insomnia is not a problem, naps may reduce stress and fatigue and improve your mood and alertness.

My past experience with naps:

I ☐ am ☐ am not a good candidate for daytime naps because:

_____

_____

_____

_____

_____

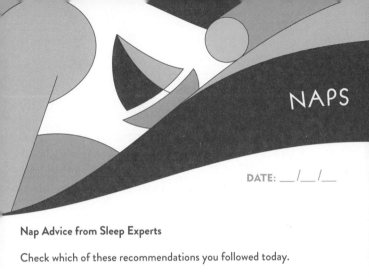

DATE: __ / __ / __

Nap Advice from Sleep Experts

Check which of these recommendations you followed today.

☐ Take your nap before 3:00 P.M. (some experts say 2:00 P.M.), or it may reduce your sleep drive and interfere with your sleep at night.

☐ Nap for no longer than 20 minutes so that you do not enter the deep stages of sleep. A too-long nap may cause sleep inertia or grogginess for the first hour after you wake up.

☐ Take your nap in a quiet, dark place, with a comfortable temperature and no distractions.

☐ Allow time to wake up fully before leaping into action.

Rate sleep in Z's: Z Z Z Z Z

A DREAM UNINTERPRETED IS LIKE A LETTER UNOPENED.

The Talmud

Explain the dream you had last night:

_____

_____

_____

_____

_____

_____

_____

DATE: ___/___/___

*Dreams are illustrations . . .
from the book your soul is
writing about you.*

Marsha Norman

Illustrate the dream you had last night:

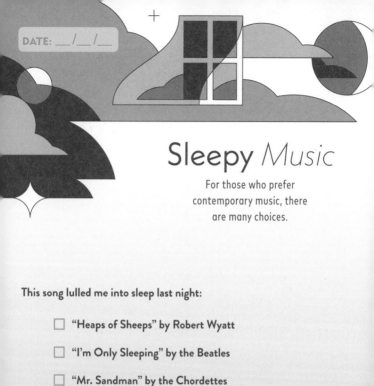

DATE: ___ / ___ / ___

Sleepy *Music*

For those who prefer
contemporary music, there
are many choices.

This song lulled me into sleep last night:

☐ "Heaps of Sheeps" by Robert Wyatt

☐ "I'm Only Sleeping" by the Beatles

☐ "Mr. Sandman" by the Chordettes

☐ "In My Room" by the Beach Boys

☐ *Sleeping Tapes* by Jeff Bridges (spoken word

and ambient music)

☐ _____

other

Let's give the humble lullaby some love. And maybe even decide it isn't so humble after all. Entire societies were raised on these songs.

Ted Gioia

A humble lullaby that still puts me to sleep:

_____

_____

_____

_____

_____

THE BEST BRIDGE
BETWEEN
DESPAIR AND
HOPE IS A GOOD
NIGHT'S SLEEP.

E. Joseph Cossman

DATE: __/__/__

SLEEP

_____   _____
DESPAIR   HOPE

DATE: __/__/__

SLEEP

_____   _____
DESPAIR   HOPE

O bed! O bed! Delicious bed! That heaven upon earth to the weary head.

Thomas Hood

Draw your delicious bed.

The days when a princess was too delicate to sleep on a mattress with a pea under it are long gone.

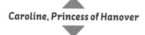

Caroline, Princess of Hanover

Last night I was not too delicate to sleep on _____.

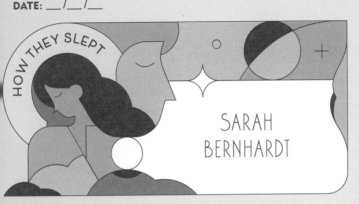

HOW THEY SLEPT

SARAH
BERNHARDT

The French actress Sarah Bernhardt said that she slept best in a coffin. She kept one in her bedroom and, most famously, traveled with a coffin, where she claimed to sleep. A widely circulated photo shows a peaceful Bernhardt lying in a coffin, eyes closed and body draped with flowers.

The strangest place I ever slept:

_____

_____

_____

_____

_____

Whenever I can't sleep, I like to lie in the darkness and pretend I've been assassinated. I've found this is the best way to get comfortable. I imagine I'm in the coffin at my funeral, and people from my past are walking by my corpse and making comments about my demise.

Chuck Klosterman

Last night, when I couldn't sleep, I imagined this bizarre scene:

_____

_____

_____

_____

_____

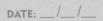

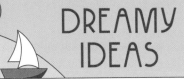

DREAMY IDEAS

Mattress for Me

Does your mattress sag or dip? Do you wake up with aches and pains? If so, you may need a new mattress. Product raters offer useful specifics, but in truth you are the best mattress tester of all. Spend as long as a half hour lying on each candidate in your favorite sleep position before making a choice. Your ideal mattress will be firm enough to support your spine and hold your body straight, but soft enough not to push against your heavy or bony parts (shoulder, hips, knees).

This is my ideal mattress:

_____

(Mattresses) . . . are large, friendly, pocket-sprung creatures that live quiet private lives in the marshes of Sqornshellous Zeta.

Douglas Adams

Weirdest mattress I have ☐ slept ☐ tossed and turned on:

_____

_____

_____

_____

_____

DATE: ___ / ___ / ___

MUSIC THAT SWEPT AWAY MY CARES LAST NIGHT:

_____

_____

_____

_____

_____

_____

DATE: ___ / ___ / ___

_____ THAT SWEPT AWAY MY CARES LAST NIGHT:

_____

_____

_____

_____

_____

_____

AND THE NIGHT SHALL
BE FILLED WITH MUSIC,
AND THE CARES, THAT
INFEST THE DAY,
SHALL FOLD THEIR
TENTS, LIKE THE ARABS,
AND AS SILENTLY
STEAL AWAY.

Henry Wadsworth Longfellow

DATE: __ / __ / __

Care-charmer Sleep, son of the sable Night.

Samuel Daniel

Care charmed away as I slept last night:

_____

_____

_____

_____

_____

If you can't sleep, then get up and do something instead of lying there worrying. It's the worry that gets you, not the lack of sleep.

Dale Carnegie

What I did instead of lying in bed worrying last night:

_____

_____

_____

_____

_____

QUIZ Z Z Z Z Z

Sleep Numbers

Circle the correct number to fill in the blank.

1. Adults need _____ or more hours of sleep every night for the
   (6 7 8)

   greatest health and well-being.

2. _____ of U.S. adults report getting less than
   (Half One-third One-quarter)

   the recommended amount of sleep each night.

3. For a 40-year-old, it takes _____ minutes to fall asleep.
   (7 17 27)

4. The ideal length of a nap is _____ minutes.
   (20 40 60)

5. The ideal temperature for sleep is _____.
   (54–60°F 60–67°F 67–72°F)

6. About _____ percent of people snore at least occasionally.
   (15 25 45)

Facts do not cease to exist because they are ignored.

Aldous Huxley

A fact on the opposite page I will not ignore:

_____

_____

How I will change my behavior:

_____

_____

*When you're lying awake
with a dismal headache,
and repose is taboo'd by anxiety,
I conceive you may use any
language you choose to indulge
in without impropriety.*

W. S. Gilbert

Last night, when I couldn't sleep, I ☐ sang ☐ swore

☐ recited _____.

This ☐ did ☐ did not help me sleep.

Don't fight with your pillow, but lay down your head. And kick every worriment out of the bed.

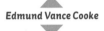

Edmund Vance Cooke

How I kicked the worriment out of my bed last night:

_____

_____

_____

_____

_____

HIS SLEEP WAS A SENSUOUS GLUTTONY OF OBLIVION.

P. D. James

DATE: ___/___/___

LAST NIGHT I DIDN'T WORRY ABOUT MY ☐ FINANCES

☐ **LOVE LIFE** ☐ _____.

other

DATE: ___/___/___

LAST NIGHT I DIDN'T WORRY ABOUT ALL THIS WORK, WHICH I HAVE TO DO TODAY:

_____

_____

_____

_____

_____

_____

DATE: ___ /___ /___

I have thought of a pulley to raise me gradually; but that
would give me pain, as it would counteract my natural
inclination. I would have something that can dissipate the
inertia and give elasticity to the muscles. We can heat the
body, we can cool it; we can give it tension or relaxation;
and surely it is possible to bring it into a state in which
rising from bed will not be a pain.

▲
Samuel Johnson
▼

Describe a device that would raise you gradually and painlessly from bed:

_____

_____

_____

_____

_____

_____

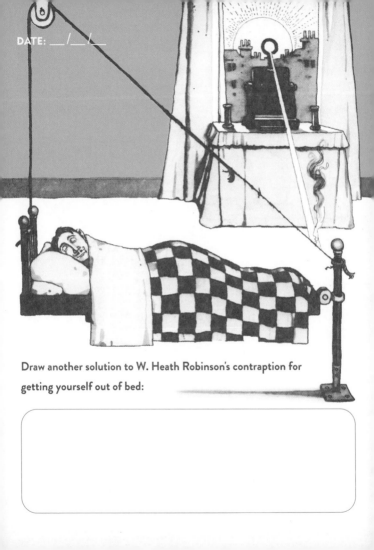

DATE: ___/___/___

Draw another solution to W. Heath Robinson's contraption for getting yourself out of bed:

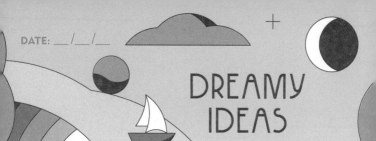

DREAMY IDEAS

Alarm Clock

Put the alarm clock far away from the bed or turn it around so that you don't see the numbers. Being able to check the time all night keeps you from sleeping. Also, avoid the snooze button. The extra time disrupts restorative sleep and can make you groggy.

Last night:

☐ I hid the clock.

☐ I didn't use the snooze button.

Rate sleep in Z's: Z Z Z Z Z

DATE: __ /__ /__

I saw something stupid in the paper today—a new alarm clock that makes no noise. It's for people who don't like loud noises. Instead, it slowly hits you with light and gets brighter and brighter until you wake up. I already have one of those . . . it's called a window.

Jay Leno

What I could use to wake up instead of an alarm clock:

_____

_____

_____

_____

_____

DATE: __ / __ / __

I am worn to a raveling.

Beatrix Potter

What wore me out yesterday:

_____

_____

_____

_____

_____

DATE: __ / __ / __

I could lay my head on a piece of lead

And imagine it was a springy bed

'Cause I'm sleepy, sleepy.

Cat Stevens

Where I fell asleep last night because I was so sleepy, sleepy:

_____

_____

_____

_____

_____

DATE: __ / __ / __

LAST NIGHT'S DREAM OF A CURRENT UNSOLVED PROBLEM AND POSSIBLE SOLUTION:

_____

_____

_____

_____

_____

DATE: __ / __ / __

LAST NIGHT'S DREAM OF A FUTURE UNSOLVED PROBLEM AND POSSIBLE SOLUTION:

_____

_____

_____

_____

_____

DREAMS REFLECT
CURRENT AND FUTURE
UNSOLVED PROBLEMS
AND REHEARSE THEIR
POSSIBLE SOLUTIONS.

Alfred Adler

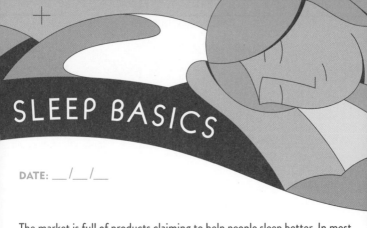

SLEEP BASICS

DATE: __ / __ / __

The market is full of products claiming to help people sleep better. In most cases, you are the best judge of what will work for you. Research, read reviews, try out different brands, and record your top choices.

Products to control temperature, noise, and darkness:

cooling mattress / sheets: _____

thick rug pad: _____

noise / white-noise machine: _____

phone noise apps: _____

earplugs / headphones: _____

blackout curtains / shades: _____

weather stripping / blackout tape: _____

sleep mask: _____

blue-light block / dimmer: _____

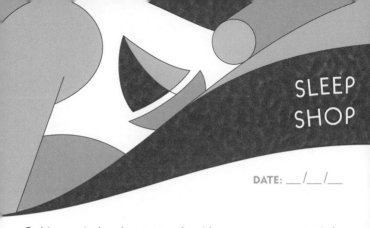

SLEEP
SHOP

DATE: ___/___/___

Bedtime stories have become popular with grownups as a way to wind down for sleep. Available as podcasts and on meditation and mindfulness apps, they include retold classics, travel tales, whispered stories, and "boring" stories, such as *Wild Flowers Worth Knowing*. Some experts believe that these stories can distract more effectively from the day's concerns than white noise or even meditation. The best ones are absorbing but not overstimulating, have comforting background music, and are told in a soothing, slow-paced voice.

I listened to this bedtime story last night:

_____

_____

_____

Rate sleep in Z's: Z Z Z Z Z

One hour's sleep before midnight is worth three after.

George Herbert

☐ I went to bed earlier than usual last night.

Rate sleep in Z's: Z Z Z Z Z

Would you have a settled head,
You must early go to bed;
I tell you, and I tell 't again,
You must be in bed by ten.

Nicholas Culpeper

I went to bed earlier than usual last night: _____:_____ ___.M.

I ☐ do ☐ do not have a settled head this morning.

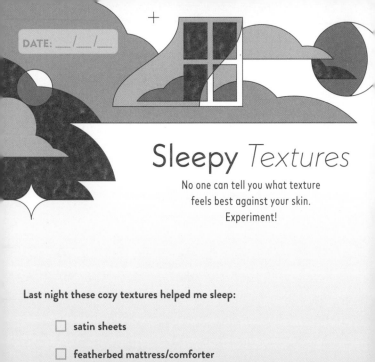

Sleepy *Textures*

No one can tell you what texture
feels best against your skin.
Experiment!

Last night these cozy textures helped me sleep:

☐ satin sheets

☐ featherbed mattress/comforter

☐ silk nightclothes

☐ flannel pajamas

☐ cashmere blanket

☐ _____

other

DATE: __ / __ / __

I PERFECTLY FEEL, EVEN AT MY FINGER'S END.

John Heywood

What felt coziest to my fingertips last night:

_____

_____

_____

_____

_____

WHEN FORCED
TO CHOOSE,
I WILL NOT TRADE
EVEN A NIGHT'S
SLEEP FOR THE
CHANCE OF
EXTRA PROFITS.

Warren Buffett

DATE: ___ / ___ / ___

I'M GLAD I DID NOT GIVE UP SLEEP TO DO THIS:

_____

_____

_____

_____

_____

_____

DATE: ___ / ___ / ___

I'M SORRY I GAVE UP SLEEP TO DO THIS:

_____

_____

_____

_____

_____

_____

How do people go to sleep? I'm afraid I've lost the knack. I might try busting myself smartly over the temple with the night-light. I might repeat to myself, slowly and soothingly, a list of quotations beautiful from minds profound; if I can remember any of the damn things.

Dorothy Parker

An insomnia cure I tried in desperation last night:

_____

_____

Rate sleep in Z's: Z Z Z Z Z

If, my dear, you seek to slumber,
Count of stars an endless number;
If you still continue wakeful,
Count the drops that make a lakeful;
Then, if vigilance yet above you
Hover, count the times I love you;
And if slumber still repel you,
Count the times I do not tell you.

Franklin P. Adams

I counted _____ to put me to sleep last night.

Rate sleep in Z's: Z Z Z Z Z

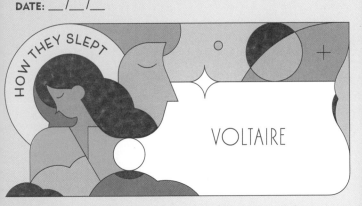

HOW THEY SLEPT

VOLTAIRE

The French writer Voltaire slept only 4 hours each night, and he loved coffee. He was known to drink up to 40 cups a day.

Before bed last night I drank:

☐ hot toddy

☐ herbal tea

☐ warm milk

☐ red wine

☐ coffee

☐ _____
other

I slept ☐ more than 4 hours ☐ less than 4 hours.

Coffee is a beverage that puts one to sleep when not drank.

Alphonse Allais

I avoided these beverages before bed last night, as sleep experts recommend:

☐ wine

☐ beer

☐ spirits

☐ coffee

☐ _____
      other

Rate sleep in Z's: Z Z Z Z Z

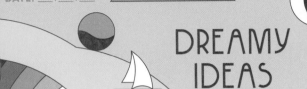

DREAMY IDEAS

Catching Up on Sleep

It is difficult to make up for lost sleep. According to a recent study, it takes 4 days to fully recover from 1 hour of lost sleep.

I lost _____ hours of sleep last night. I should be

recovered by _____.

You know it's a bad case when the only way you can catch up on your sleep is to get unconscious.

Val McDermid

I am sleep-deprived because of ☐ too much work

☐ too much play

☐ too much worry

☐ _____
other

How I plan to get back on track:

_____

DATE: ___/___/___

TODAY'S GOOD DEED FOR SOMEONE DEAR THAT SMOOTHED MY PILLOW TONIGHT:

_____

_____

_____

_____

_____

DATE: ___/___/___

TODAY'S GOOD DEED FOR SOMEONE I DON'T KNOW THAT SMOOTHED MY PILLOW TONIGHT:

_____

_____

_____

_____

_____

I pillowed
myself in
goodness
and slept
righteously.

Maya Angelou

DATE: __ / __ / __

I am convinced that a light supper, a good night's sleep, and a fine morning, have sometimes made a hero of the same man, who, by an indigestion, a restless night, and a rainy morning, would have proved a coward.

Lord Chesterfield

I had a ☐ light supper ☐ good night's sleep ☐ fine morning.

How I was a ☐ hero ☐ coward today:

_____

_____

_____

_____

I love sleep because it is both pleasant and safe to use.

Fran Lebowitz

I love sleep because:

_____

_____

_____

_____

_____

QUIZ z z z z z

My Way

Although scientists make general rules based on research, each individual is different. If the general rule doesn't work for you, pay attention to your own body.

Check the general rules you can break and still get a good night's sleep:

☐ sleep _____ ☐ more ☐ less than the time
             hours/minutes
   recommended for my age

☐ nap later than 3:00 P.M.

☐ read an engaging book in bed, right before sleep

☐ watch a video right before sleep

☐ drink a caffeinated beverage after supper

☐ exercise near bedtime

☐ fall asleep puzzling over a work problem

Think what a better world it would be if we all, the whole world, had cookies and milk about three o'clock every afternoon and then lay down on our blankets for a nap.

Barbara Jordan

Why the world seemed better after my cozy nap today at _____.M.:

_____

_____

_____

_____

_____

The armored cars of dreams,
contrived to let us do
so many a dangerous thing.

Elizabeth Bishop

Something dangerous I did in my dream last night:

_____

_____

_____

_____

_____

DATE: __ /__ /__

Dreaming permits each and every one of us to be quietly and safely insane every night of the week.

William Dement

Something insane I did in my dream last night:

_____

_____

_____

_____

_____

I SLEEP EACH NIGHT
A LITTLE BETTER,
A LITTLE MORE
CONFIDENTLY, BECAUSE
LYNDON JOHNSON
IS MY PRESIDENT.

Jack Valenti

DATE: __ / __ / __

I SLEEP EACH NIGHT A LITTLE BETTER BECAUSE _____

public reason

_____

_____

_____

_____

_____

_____

DATE: __ / __ / __

I SLEEP EACH NIGHT A LITTLE BETTER BECAUSE _____

personal reason

_____

_____

_____

_____

_____

DATE: __/__/__

A birdie with a yellow bill
Hopped upon the window sill,
Cocked his shining eye and
   said:
"Ain't you 'shamed, you
   sleepy-head."

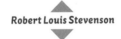

Robert Louis Stevenson

☐ This morning, deferring to the experts, I got up from bed on
schedule.

Rate sleep in Z's: **Z Z Z Z Z**

'Tis the voice of the sluggard—I heard him complain,
"You have waked me too soon, I must slumber again."
As the door on its hinges, so he on his bed,
Turns his sides, and his shoulders, and his heavy head.

Isaac Watts

☐ This morning, defying the experts, I turned over and went back to sleep.

Rate sleep in Z's: Z Z Z Z Z

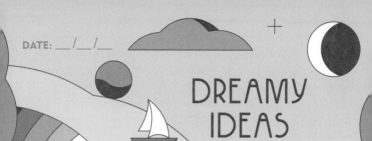

DREAMY IDEAS

Strategies for a Worry-free Sleep

Check a new strategy that you will try tonight or tried last night.

☐ Write all your worries on a piece of paper. Then crumple it up and throw it away.

☐ Write each worry on a separate card; sort them into categories (e.g., finances, relationships), then prioritize. Write a solution for each worry. If none exists, write that.

☐ Make a to-do list for the next day. This will be a relief, should you awaken in a panic.

Rate sleep in Z's: Z Z Z Z Z

DATE: __ /__ /__

It helps to write down half a dozen things which are worrying me. Two of them, say, disappear; about two, nothing can be done, so it's no use worrying; and two perhaps can be settled.

Winston Churchill

My worries today:

1. _____   4. _____

2. _____   5. _____

3. _____   6. _____

Put an X by worries that will probably disappear.

Put a Y by worries that you can do nothing about.

Put a Z by worries that perhaps can be settled.

Daytime sleep is a cursed slumber from which one wakes in despair.

Iris Murdoch

Time and length of my nap today:

_____

_____

_____

_____

Afterward I felt ☐ desperate   ☐ refreshed.

Let me tell you about the nap. It's absolutely fantastic. . . . The best part of it is that when you wake up, for the first 15 seconds, you have no idea where you are. You're just alive. That's all you know. And it's bliss.

Philip Roth

How I felt when I woke up from my nap today:

_____

_____

_____

_____

_____

DATE: ___ / ___ / ___

DRAW YOURSELF ROUNDED WITH LAST NIGHT'S SLEEP:

DATE: ___ / ___ / ___

DRAW YOURSELF JAGGED FROM LAST NIGHT'S LACK OF SLEEP:

We are
such stuff
As dreams are
made on, and
our little life
Is rounded
with a sleep.

William Shakespeare

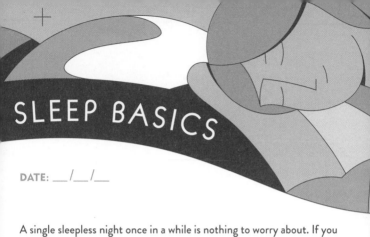

SLEEP BASICS

DATE: ___/___/___

A single sleepless night once in a while is nothing to worry about. If you often have trouble getting to sleep or staying asleep, however, even after adopting the healthy sleep habits recommended in this book, you should consider consulting a specialist. Ask your doctor for a referral or use the directory of the American Academy of Sleep Medicine, which lists accredited sleep clinics nationwide (sleepeducation.org).

Use this calendar to track the nights you have insomnia.

Start date:

___/___/___

Finish date:

___/___/___

SUN	MON	TUE	WED	THU	FRI	SAT

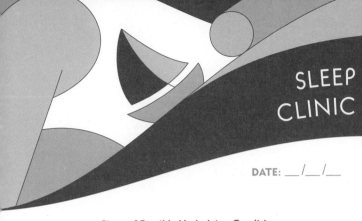

Signs of Possible Underlying Conditions

The major sleep disorders, according to the CDC, are chronic insomnia, narcolepsy, restless legs syndrome, and sleep apnea. These should be diagnosed by a health care provider. When the source is anxiety, cognitive behavioral therapy (CBT) is often recommended.

Check any symptoms you are experiencing:

- ☐ regular problem getting to sleep or staying asleep

- ☐ unexplained excessive daytime sleepiness

- ☐ reports from a bed partner that you may be having trouble breathing in your sleep—not snoring, but gasping or snorting

- ☐ frequent leg twitches or unpleasant creeping sensations in the legs or other movements during sleep

DATE: ___ / ___ / ___

The happiest part of a man's life is what he passes lying awake in bed in the morning.

Samuel Johnson

How I passed my time in bed this morning:

_____

_____

_____

_____

There is no sunrise so beautiful that it is worth waking me up to see.

Mindy Kaling

What time I got up this morning/afternoon:

_____

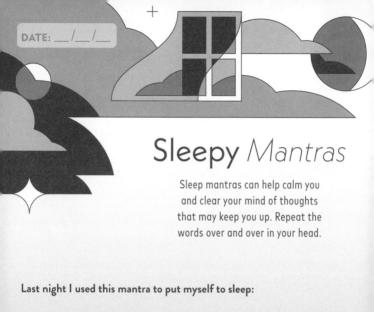

DATE: ___/___/___

Sleepy *Mantras*

Sleep mantras can help calm you
and clear your mind of thoughts
that may keep you up. Repeat the
words over and over in your head.

Last night I used this mantra to put myself to sleep:

☐ I welcome sleep.

☐ I am calm and still.

☐ I make peace with time.

☐ I release this day.

☐ I embrace my dreams.

☐ _____.
other

Rate sleep in Z's: Z Z Z Z Z

DATE: __/__/__

A ruffled mind makes a restless pillow.

Charlotte Brontë

Words that unruffled my mind last night:

_____

_____

_____

_____

_____

DATE: ___ / ___ / ___

☐ LAST NIGHT THE GOD OF SLEEP CALMED MY MIND AND PUT MY CARES TO FLIGHT.

DATE: ___ / ___ / ___

☐ LAST NIGHT THE GOD OF SLEEP SOOTHED MY WEARY LIMBS AND REFRESHED THEM FOR THEIR TOIL.

O SLEEP, IN WHOM ALL
THINGS FIND REST, MOST
PEACEFUL OF THE GODS,
YOU WHO CALM THE MIND,
PUT CARES TO FLIGHT,
SOOTHE LIMBS WEARIED BY
HARSH TASKS AND REFRESH
THEM FOR THEIR TOIL.

Ovid

I love the silent hour of night,

For blissful dreams may then arise,

Revealing to my charmed sight

What may not bless my waking eyes!

Anne Brontë

What I see in the silent hour of night:

_____

_____

_____

_____

_____

*Elected Silence, sing
   to me
And beat upon my
   whorlèd ear*

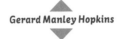

Gerard Manley Hopkins

What I hear in the silence of the night:

_____

_____

_____

_____

_____

Ninety-nine zillion,
Nine trillion and two
Creatures are sleeping!
So . . .
How about you?

Dr. Seuss

How about you?

_____

_____

_____

_____

_____

SLEEP SURVEY

Before filling out this survey, review your sleep ratings at the bottoms of the pages throughout this book.

Number of hours I sleep at night: _____

    Bedtime: _____

    Wake time: _____

Naps: ☐ yes ☐ no

    How many? _____

    Average length: _____

Dinner time: _____

Unplug time: _____

Ways I relax before sleep:

_____

How well I sleep (rate in Z's): Z Z Z Z

Compare this to the survey you took at the beginning of this book:

_____

_____

_____

_____

_____

ISBN 978-0-593-23656-7

Printed in Malaysia

Conceived and compiled by Dian G. Smith and Robie Rogge

Editor: Lindley Boegehold
Designer: Annalisa Sheldahl
Production Editor: Abby Oladipo
Production Manager: Kelli Tokos
Compositors: Nick Patton and DIX Type
Copy Editor: Alison Hagge
Illustrator: Calvin Sprague

10 9 8 7 6 5 4 3 2 1

First Edition